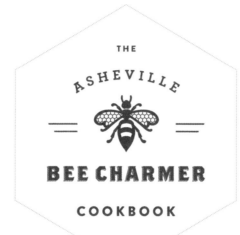

THE

ASHEVILLE

BEE CHARMER

COOKBOOK

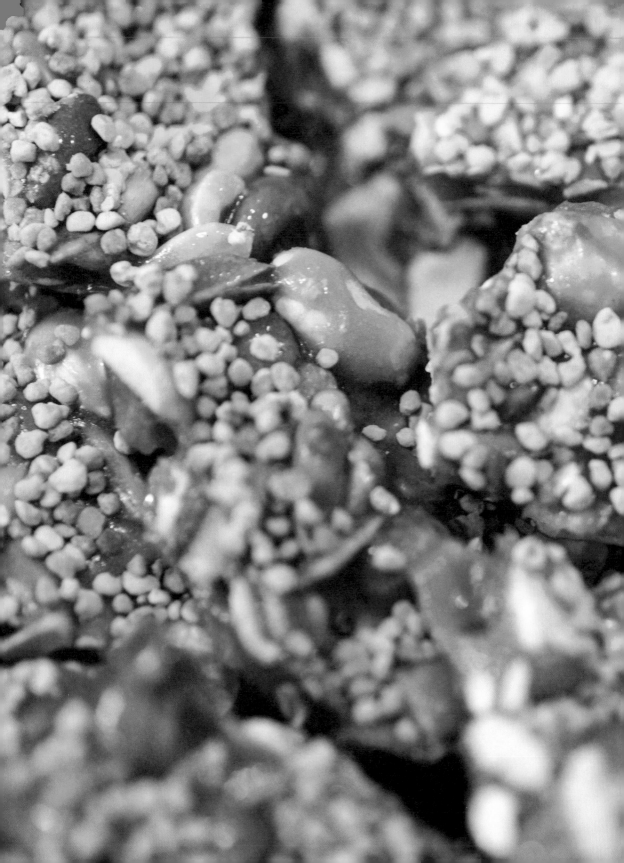

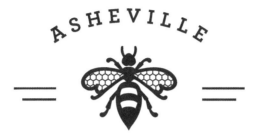

THE
ASHEVILLE
BEE CHARMER
COOKBOOK

Sweet *and* Savory Recipes INSPIRED BY 28 Honey Varietals *and* Blends

CARRIE SCHLOSS

FOREWORD BY Jillian Kelly and Kim Allen

PHOTOGRAPHY BY Angela B. Garbot

SURREY BOOKS

AN AGATE IMPRINT

CHICAGO

Printed in China

Photography by Angela B. Garbot
Cover illustration by Antonina Sharafutdinova (iStock.com/Nujtmom)

Library of Congress Cataloging-in-Publication Data

Names: Schloss, Carrie, author. | Asheville Bee Charmer, author.
Title: The Asheville Bee Charmer cookbook : sweet and savory recipes inspired
  by 28 honey varietals and blends / Carrie Schloss ; foreword by Jillian
  Kelly and Kim Allen ; photography by Angela B. Garbot.
Description: Chicago : Surrey Books, an Agate imprint, [2017] | Includes
  index.
Identifiers: LCCN 2017003904 (print) | LCCN 2017008898 (ebook) | ISBN
  9781572842281 (pbk.) | ISBN 1572842288 (pbk.) | ISBN 9781572848016 (ebook)
  | ISBN 1572848014 (ebook)
Subjects: LCSH: Cooking (Honey) | Honey. | LCGFT: Cookbooks.
Classification: LCC TX767.H7 S34 2017 (print) | LCC TX767.H7 (ebook) | DDC
  641.6/8--dc23
LC record available at https://lccn.loc.gov/2017003904

10 9 8 7 6 5 4 3 2 1   17 18 19 20 21

Surrey Books is an imprint of Agate Publishing. Agate books are available in bulk at discount prices. For more information, visit agatepublishing.com.

To my mom, Rosita Schloss, who let me start cooking for our family when I was around ten or eleven years old, has always encouraged me to follow my own path and achieve my dreams no matter where that may lead, and is always an enthusiastic taste tester.

Contents

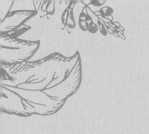

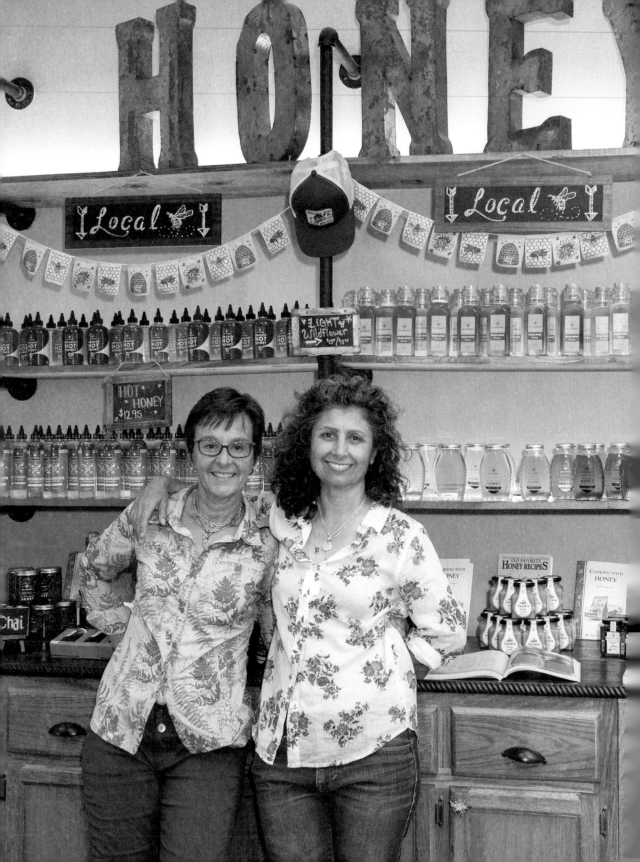

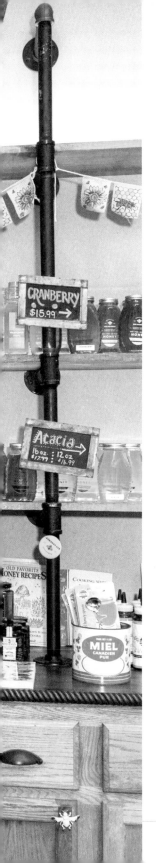

Foreword

AFTER FALLING IN LOVE WITH ASHEVILLE over ten years of frequent visits, we decided it was time to embrace a healthier and slower-paced lifestyle by changing "hives" and moving to our dream city a few years ago. During the years before our move, we also began changing our diet by choosing farmers' markets and organic food over more traditional supermarkets and processed foods. Wanting to replace white refined sugar with something healthier, we began experimenting with a number of alternative sweeteners and found honey to be the natural, clear choice for our kitchen. Learning about different types of honey became a passion for us. And the more we learned about all the natural benefits that honey and bees provide, the more our fascination with bees grew, eventually leading us to take beekeeping classes.

We opened our store in 2014 as a way to connect with the local community and share our passion about honey and bees with our customers. The Asheville Bee Charmer is more than just a honey store—it's an experience that hits all your senses the moment you walk into our hive. We create an atmosphere of curiosity that invites our customers to participate and appreciate. Our expert bee-ristas are on hand to make the honey-tasting bar experience a joyful and educational one.

Since our move, we also have become beekeepers. We adopted many beautiful, magical, and amazing bees and searched to find a healthy environment where they could live and thrive. Through connections from our beekeeping club, those locations found us. Our bees reside on a local farm, as well as private land surrounded by tulip poplar, locust trees, and many other pollinator-friendly plants. Both locations provide the four seasons for our honeybees. In addition to our excitement about our honey production, soon after we opened, the buzz was in the air about the local honey store in western North Carolina. Many beekeepers from both our local beekeeping club and beyond Asheville have connected with us over their love of beekeeping. Although we do carry a few select honeys from artisan producers worldwide, the majority of our honey is sourced from small-batch, ethical, regional-based local and artisan honey producers. This gives us the feeling of community that we have been looking for in a smaller town surrounded by mountains and nature. And we actively work on some smaller projects to help raise money for Bee City USA and the Center for Honeybee Research here in Asheville.

> Our bees reside on a local farm, as well as private land surrounded by tulip poplar, locust trees, and many other pollinator-friendly plants.

It feels like the pieces to this magical life keep falling into place at the right time, as our business has expanded and grown in a direction we never had dreamed possible. Little did we know that a visit from Carrie would turn into this beautiful project, which she created from her knowledge of cooking with honey and her boundless vision for delicious edible creations. Kim and Carrie's friendship goes back to their college days and was built upon their mutual love of food and travel. Through the years, we have been to Carrie's house for dinner many times. We always look forward to those invitations because we have always been impressed with the meals she prepares and the flavor combinations she uses to provide a mouthwatering culinary experience.

Last year, Carrie arrived in Asheville to visit, armed with a list of restaurants she wanted to go to in order to experience Asheville's unique food culture. She came to the store to taste honey, and while she was at the honey bar, you could already see the wheels turning as to how she would use the different honeys in various dishes. Her refined palate for the variety of flavors was inspiring. It's not every day one gets to sit and taste at least 40 different varieties of honey (we actually did this over a couple of days). Many Asheville food tours stop at the Asheville Bee Charmer. Someone always asks how to use the different types of honey in their cooking. Since we always experiment with honey ourselves, we offer up what we have tried. During her visit, Carrie happened to be tasting honey when one of the food tours stopped by. When the inevitable question arose, she chimed right in and offered up amazing ideas.

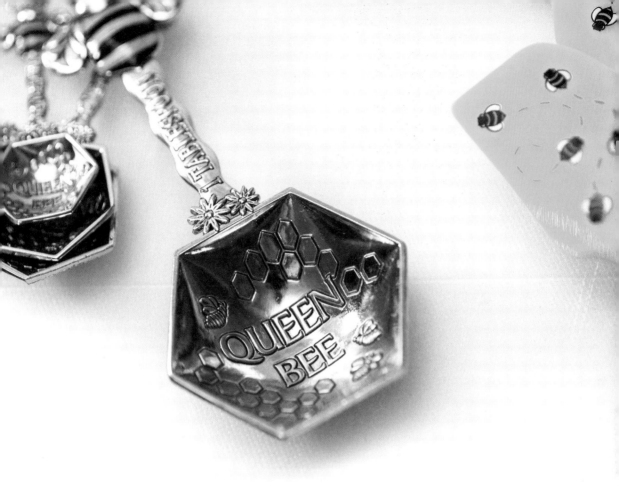

Since we opened our store, we have often been asked when we would write a honey cookbook. We didn't think we could write one ourselves, but after seeing Carrie in action at the honey bar, we thought she could bring the project to fruition. Knowing how focused and dedicated she is, we were sure she would create everyday recipes that would be easy and enjoyable to make with clear and straightforward directions—and that's exactly what *The Asheville Bee Charmer Cookbook* contains. Her use of honey brings a new twist to recipes and adds another level of flavor to food in a unique way. We believe her creative cooking ideas will inspire each reader to experiment with the wide variety of honey flavors available here in the United States and abroad. We hope you'll enjoy this journey of honey and cooking as much as we have; we sampled a lot of the recipes in this book! And the next time you pass through Asheville, we'll have a stool waiting for you at the honey bar.

—Jillian Kelly and Kim Allen

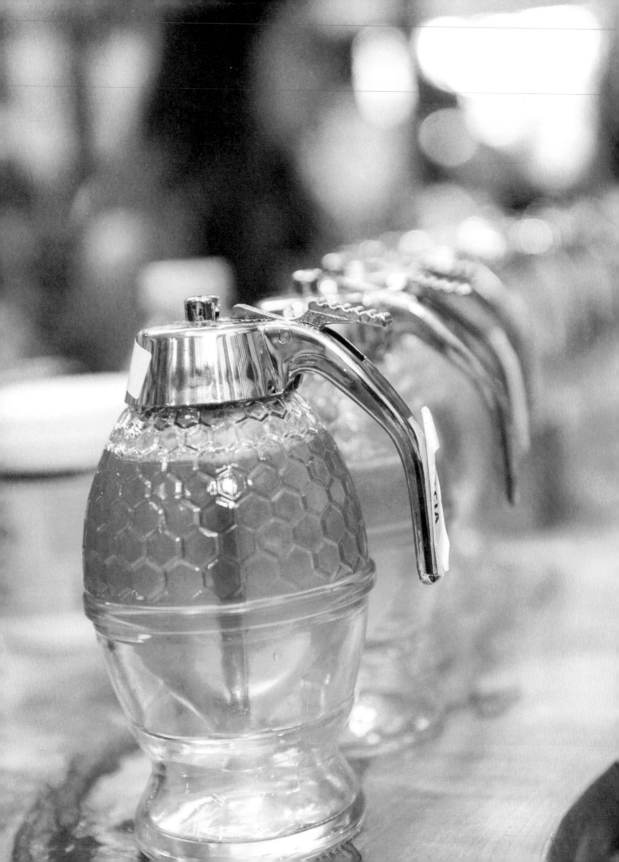

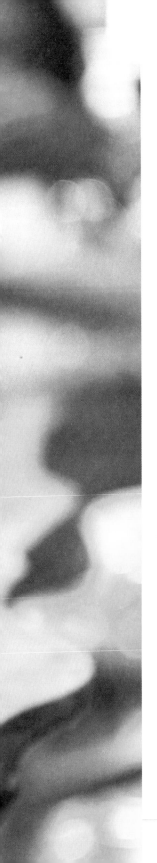

Introduction

IF YOU ASK SOMEONE ABOUT HONEY, you usually get one of three responses: (1) it's the plastic bear sold in the supermarket, (2) its primary use is in tea or a hot toddy when someone's sick, or (3) it tastes really sweet. All of those statements may be true, but what many don't realize is that the world of honey is much larger than the little bear on the shelf—and the taste of honey is much more complex than merely being "sweet." When I told friends I was writing a cookbook for the Asheville Bee Charmer, there was an immediate assumption that it was merely a dessert cookbook. When I explained that I was using 28 varietals of honey, I often received a puzzled look and a comment about how they didn't realize there were that many types of honey.

I completely understand both responses. Growing up, most of the honey I tasted and used was either a wildflower or clover blend. Through my career as a chef, my exposure to local Illinois farmers, and my work on the board of Slow Food Chicago, I learned of the many local artisanal honey producers in my area, and my honey palate started to expand. Although there are a small number of unique varieties available, the majority of honey available in my region is wildflower blends from distinct neighborhoods. But, according to the National Honey Board, there are over 300 unique or monofloral honey varietals (which means the honey has a distinctive flavor as it is mostly made from the nectar of one kind of plant) in the United States. In fact, it is estimated that there are thousands of unique honey varietals worldwide.

Artisanal honey harvests are very short, seasonal, and limited in yield. When bees bring nectar back to the hive to put in the honeycomb, they also bring pollen. As worker bees pack this pollen, it becomes bee pollen. In large batch production, bee pollen frequently gets filtered out of the "honey." The food safety divisions of the World Health Organization, the European Commission, and other worldwide organizations have determined that without pollen, there is no way to determine whether honey has come from legitimate and safe sources. In the United States, the Food and Drug Administration says that any product that's been ultra-filtered and no longer contains pollen isn't actually honey. Because of these factors, it's important to understand, as you should with other types of food that you buy, where the product comes from and how it was processed. There are currently no labeling laws for honey, so what is labeled as "honey" can be anything from 100-percent pure honey containing pollen, to honey mixed with sugar and/or corn syrup, to a mixture of honeys containing no pollen.

A varietal is a distinct type of honey created from the nectar of a specific flower source visited by the honeybee.

When I first visited the Queen Bees, Kim and Jill, at their small honey store, the Asheville Bee Charmer, I expected to be wowed by their selection of about 50 unique honey varietals, some locally sourced and some from small artisanal producers worldwide, as well as their other honey- and bee-related products. What I didn't expect was the full engagement of most of my senses as soon as I walked through the door. The first thing you notice is the wall of honey. I knew honey ranged in color; I had seen lighter colored early-harvest honey

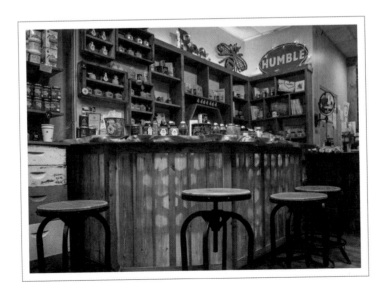

and darker colored late-harvest honey, but I wasn't really prepared for the expansive breadth of colors and hues of the unique honey varietals. I saw everything from almost translucent honey to honey so dark it looked like molasses.

If you've ever visited the store, you know that your senses of smell, taste, and touch also get a workout. In one corner sits the honey bar, where you can smell and taste all 50 honey varietals they sell. Most of the honey I had previously smelled had a slightly floral scent because it was primarily of the wildflower or clover varietals. I wasn't prepared to smell everything from citrus to dirty socks as I made my way through the assortment of honey. Taste, so linked with aroma, is a similar story. In general, early-harvest honey tends to be milder in flavor and late-harvest honey tends to be bolder in flavor, but depending on the honey, flavor notes can range from familiar floral to toasted marshmallows to leather. Additionally, some varietals are sweeter than others, which is related to the ratio of glucose and fructose in the honey. As for touch, it's all about mouthfeel, or the physical sensations created by the honey on your tongue, your teeth, the roof of your mouth, and even at the back of your mouth as you swallow. Most of the honey I had used in the past had a single viscosity level, but depending on the floral source, honey can be thin and pourable or thick enough to scoop with a spoon.

What struck me as I sat at the honey bar was that honey is a lot like wine. Each varietal has a unique color, aroma, taste, and mouthfeel. Additionally, like wine, each varietal is influenced by *terroir*, the set of environmental factors, such as soil conditions, weather, and temperature, which affect a plant during its growth cycle and contribute to differences in flavor and aroma. For example, you can taste three different clover honeys that were each produced in a different location, and discover that each one has a slightly different aroma, color, and taste, depending on the location's terroir—just like a chardonnay produced in northern California will have different characteristics than one produced in central California or one produced in France. A varietal from the same location or field can also have a different taste from year to year depending on weather conditions; think of the differences between a specific vineyard's wines from year to year.

The Honey and Pollination Center at the Robert Mondavi Institute for Wine and Food Science at UC Davis has created a honey flavor wheel, which breaks down taste into basic flavor categories such as fruity, floral, herbaceous, woody, chemical, animal, nutty, spicy, caramel, earthy, and microbiological. Within those categories the flavors are further broken down into more specific categories. For example, the fruity category includes flavor notes such as berry, citrus, dried fruit, tree fruit, and tropical fruit. It is available online and is a great tool to use when tasting to help increase your honey vocabulary.

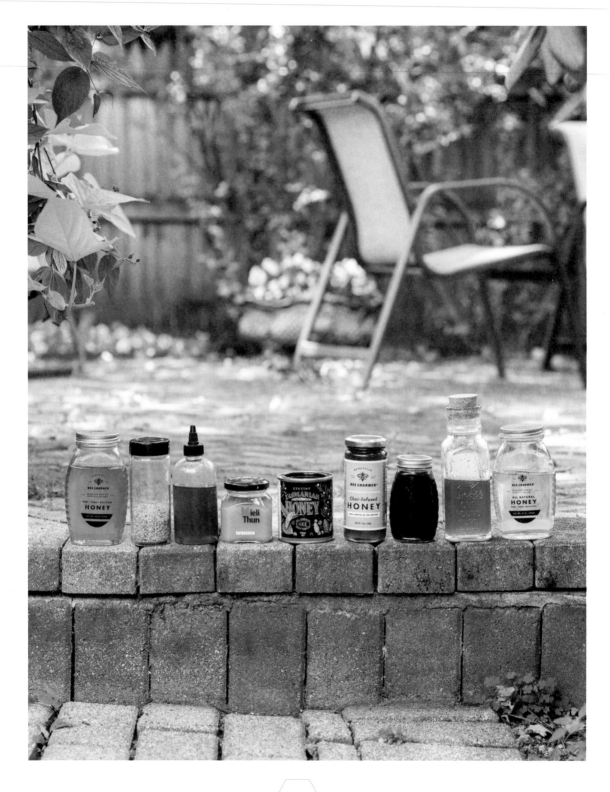

THE HONEY VARIETALS IN THIS BOOK

Here, I have provided a simple guide to the varietals used in the recipes in this book. It is meant to be a broad overview of the color, aroma, and taste you can expect from each varietal, along with some ideas of what foods pair well with the honey. The first seven honeys listed are proprietary blends created through infusions by the Asheville Bee Charmer, which are only available at their brick-and-mortar and online stores. The remaining blends and varietals can be purchased at the Asheville Bee Charmer and elsewhere.

ASHEVILLE BEE CHARMER BLENDS

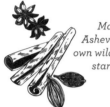

CHAI
Made by infusing the Asheville Bee Charmer's own wildflower honey with star anise, cardamom, cinnamon, ginger, and secret spices.

COLOR: dark brown

AROMA: chai spices, floral

TASTE: floral, chai spices, cinnamon, ginger

PAIRS WELL WITH: Indian food, Moroccan food, tea, squash, grilled fruit, ice cream, waffles, pancakes, apples

COCOA
Made by infusing the Asheville Bee Charmer's own wildflower honey with pure raw cacao.

COLOR: almost black

AROMA: chocolate and cocoa

TASTE: sweetened bittersweet chocolate

PAIRS WELL WITH: anything with chocolate, warm milk, warm crusty bread, fruit, waffles, pancakes

FIRECRACKER HOT
Made by infusing the Asheville Bee Charmer's own raw wildflower or clover honey with locally grown North Carolina chiles and a dash of vinegar.

COLOR: reddish hue

AROMA: chiles, warm beeswax, floral, vegetal

TASTE: sweet heat

PAIRS WELL WITH: Asian food, Mexican food, Moroccan food, chicken, salmon, steak, peaches, Greek yogurt, ice cream

GHOST PEPPER
Made by infusing the Asheville Bee Charmer's own clover honey with in-season, locally grown ghost peppers.

COLOR: straw to yellow color with buttery-yellow hue

AROMA: chiles, warm beeswax, vegetal

TASTE: sweet heat

PAIRS WELL WITH: Asian food, Mexican food, grilled cheese, braised cabbage, braised sausage

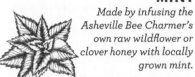

MINT

Made by infusing the Asheville Bee Charmer's own raw wildflower or clover honey with locally grown mint.

COLOR: straw to yellow color with light green hue

AROMA: floral, vegetal, grass, mint

TASTE: light spice, vegetal, mint

PAIRS WELL WITH: vinaigrettes, lamb, spring rolls, tea, fruit, ice cream

ROSEMARY

Made by infusing the Asheville Bee Charmer's own raw wildflower or clover honey with locally grown rosemary.

COLOR: straw to yellow color with light-green hue

AROMA: floral, vegetal, warm beeswax, rosemary

TASTE: light spice, vegetal, rosemary

PAIRS WELL WITH: braised dishes, savory bread pudding, roast chicken, polenta cake, lamb

SMOKIN' HOT (CHIPOTLE-INFUSED HONEY)

Made by infusing the Asheville Bee Charmer's own raw wildflower or clover honey with locally grown, applewood-smoked North Carolina chipotle chiles and a dash of vinegar.

COLOR: reddish hue

AROMA: chiles, molasses, smoke

TASTE: sweet heat, smoke, molasses

PAIRS WELL WITH: Mexican food, barbeque, ribs, chicken, steak, eggplant, corn bread, Bloody Marys

OTHER HONEY BLENDS AND VARIETALS

ACACIA

Comes from the nectar of the false acacia (black locust) tree, which grows in the eastern United States, Italy, France, Hungary, Bulgaria, Ukraine, Serbia, Romania, Canada, and China. Acacia honey has a very high fructose level, which means it is one of the few honeys in the world that won't crystallize.

COLOR: very pale, almost clear, with a lemon-white or yellow-green hue

AROMA: very slight floral, fruity, sweet almonds

TASTE: very mild taste, floral, hints of vanilla, golden raisin, currant

PAIRS WELL WITH: Asian dishes, stuffing, tomato sauce, fruit, ice cream, fresh farmer's cheese or ricotta, and strong-flavored cheeses such as aged pecorino, aged Parmigiano-Reggiano, blue cheese, or Gorgonzola

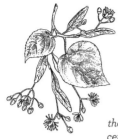

BASSWOOD

Also known as American linden honey, native to southern Canada, the Appalachians, the eastern and south central United States, France, Spain, Germany, Russia, Poland, China, Ukraine, Hungary, and the United Kingdom. It's known as "lime tree honey" in Europe.

COLOR: light to medium amber, with creamy yellow and green hues

AROMA: fresh, woody, incense, resin, caramel, buttermilk, beeswax, musty

TASTE: menthol, sage, mint, balsamic, camphor, biting aromatic flavor, candied lime zest, grapefruit, pineapple, butterscotch, crisp green melon, green banana with metallic finish, slightly citric and bitter aftertaste

PAIRS WELL WITH: sweet-and-sour foods, sweet-and-tart foods, roasted meat, roasted vegetables, bacon, guacamole, and foods cooked with sage, basil, and lemongrass

BLACKBERRY

Native to the Pacific Northwest, particularly Oregon, which is the largest producer of cultivated blackberries in the United States. It's also produced in Texas, Virginia (and elsewhere on the East Coast in the United States), Mexico, Chile, Brazil, Guatemala, the United Kingdom, New Zealand, and parts of southern and eastern Europe. This honey crystallizes very quickly.

COLOR: light amber with a burnt-orange tint if from the Pacific Northwest, creamy tint if from the East Coast

AROMA: currants, brown sugar

TASTE: floral, lemon peel, butter

PAIRS WELL WITH: fresh cheese, mascarpone, eggs, berries, citrus, salmon, ham, vanilla ice cream, sour cream pound cake

BLUEBERRY

Native to New England (particularly Maine), Michigan, Wisconsin, Oregon, New Jersey, California, Florida, and Georgia.

COLOR: light amber

AROMA: fruity

TASTE: blueberry, violet, jasmine, lemon, slightly tangy

PAIRS WELL WITH: beets, sweet-and-tart foods, fresh cheese, goat cheese, sparkling white wine, Greek yogurt, muesli, eggs, berries, lemon, pastries, venison

BUCKWHEAT

Native to Minnesota, New York, Ohio, Pennsylvania, North Dakota, South Dakota, and Wisconsin in the United States. Abroad, it's produced in eastern Canada, Poland, Romania, Ukraine, Russia, and China.

COLOR: dark brown to ebony, like molasses

AROMA: dirty socks/laundry, musty basement, malty beer, aged wood furniture

TASTE: chocolate malt balls, dark red cherries, toasted toffee, molasses

PAIRS WELL WITH: buckwheat, Asian dishes, legumes, barbeque, spiced cookies, nutty cheddar, Stilton, chocolate, pastries, chocolate hazelnut gelato

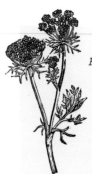

CARROT

Found wherever carrot seeds are produced. In the United States, carrot honey hails mostly from the Willamette Valley, but it can also be found in Europe, particularly in Italy.

COLOR: yellow-orange to dark amber

AROMA: sweet resin, almond extract, coconut, tanning lotion

TASTE: salty milk, caramel with a finish of bitter almonds, celery, grass, earthy, mushroom

PAIRS WELL WITH: sweet spices, black pepper, bread with fruits and nuts, root vegetables, bitter greens, duck, mushrooms

CLOVER

One of the most widely available honey varietals worldwide, particularly in Canada, the United States, Sweden, New Zealand, and China. White sweet clover is the most prevalent type of clover honey, but there are also yellow sweet clover honey and crimson clover honey. This honey crystallizes very quickly.

COLOR: varies from light white (white and yellow sweet clover) to an array of amber (crimson clover); most are a straw to yellow color with buttery-yellow or light-green hue

AROMA: light spice, floral, vegetal, warm beeswax, dry hay, grass, cinnamon, brown butter, vanilla

TASTE: mild and light with a sweet, crisp, and clean floral taste, cinnamon

PAIRS WELL WITH: Indian food, Moroccan food, lemon

CORSICAN BLOSSOM

Native to Corsica, a Mediterranean island belonging to France. Corsican blossom honey is made from the nectar of wildflowers that grow on the island, and it's the only French honey that is certified for origin and quality (appellation d'origine contrôlée, or AOC), much like many French wines.

COLOR: dark brown

AROMA: licorice, coconut, woody

TASTE: woody, caramel, cacao, dark brown sugar, sorghum, licorice

PAIRS WELL WITH: root vegetables, chocolate chip cookies, goat cheese, Parmigiano-Reggiano

CRANBERRY

Produced in Wisconsin and the Northeast United States.

COLOR: dark amber with red tint to deep red

AROMA: cranberry, floral

TASTE: tart red cranberry, cinnamon, candied fruit, brown sugar, dried plums

PAIRS WELL WITH: stuffing, Brie, kale salad, pumpkin bread, spice cake, roasted turkey, apples, dark chocolate, chamomile tea

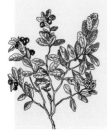

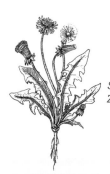

DANDELION
Native to Greece, Italy, North and South America, New Zealand, and China.

COLOR: sunshine yellow

AROMA: sulfur, ammonia, milk, wet hay, wet socks, musty

TASTE: vanilla, chamomile

PAIRS WELL WITH: endive, escarole, egg pasta, roasted or grilled pork, lemon, aromatic herbs, aged Parmigiano-Reggiano, blue cheese

FIR
Comes from the nectar of aromatic fir trees found in high-elevation forests of central Greece.

COLOR: dark amber

AROMA: pine resin, barley, smoky, burnt sugar, crème brûlée, animal scents

TASTE: malt, caramel, toasted barley, toffee, molasses

PAIRS WELL WITH: bacon, fatty cured meats, sourdough bread, fruit salad, duck, brown bread, cookies, cakes, pretzels, brittle

GINGER
Made by infusing acacia honey with raw ginger.

COLOR: straw to yellow color with buttery-yellow hue

AROMA: light spice, floral, fruity, ginger

TASTE: spice, ginger

PAIRS WELL WITH: Asian food, Moroccan food, vinaigrettes, salads, shrimp, fish

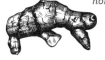

LAVENDER
Produced in southern Europe, North Africa, East Africa, the Mediterranean, southwest Asia, and France.

COLOR: light yellow, sometimes white with tinges of gold; the closer it's produced to the sea, the darker it becomes

AROMA: cat pee, floral, camphor, almond, vanilla

TASTE: light, delicate, floral, lavender, peach, slightly acidic

PAIRS WELL WITH: feta cheese, blue cheese, triple-cream cheese, apple, cabbage, walnuts

MEADOWFOAM
Produced in Oregon's Willamette Valley and the Pacific Northwest in the United States. Meadowfoam is a low-growing herbaceous winter plant. Its name refers to its appearance; at full bloom it is a solid canopy of creamy white flowers.

COLOR: light, clear amber

AROMA: vanilla

TASTE: toasted marshmallow, vanilla, caramelized custard, burnt sugar

PAIRS WELL WITH: chocolate, dessert, hot chocolate, chocolate ice cream

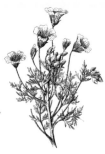

ORANGE BLOSSOM

Produced domestically in Arizona, California, Texas, and Florida, and abroad in Mexico, Brazil, Spain, and France.

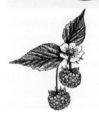

COLOR: medium amber with burnt orange, tangerine, and golden hues

AROMA: orange blossom, fresh flowers, honeysuckle, hawthorn, hyacinth, ripe yellow melon

TASTE: floral, orange, tangerine, rose, jasmine

PAIRS WELL WITH: pastries, wheat pasta, spring vegetable omelet, raw or cooked fish, duck

RASPBERRY

Produced throughout the United States.

COLOR: light amber

AROMA: floral, cocoa butter

TASTE: berry, meadow, lilac, floral

PAIRS WELL WITH: berries, pastries, fresh cheese

SAGE

Produced along the coastline and hills of California.

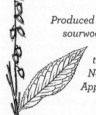

COLOR: light amber, golden raisin

AROMA: woody, roasted food, brown sugar

TASTE: beeswax, oak, toasty, smoky

PAIRS WELL WITH: stuffing, mushrooms, lamb, lasagna, apple, turkey, savory bread pudding

SOURWOOD

Produced from the nectar of the sourwood tree, also known as the lily-of-the-valley tree. It can be found in North Carolina and the Appalachian Mountains.

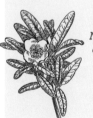

COLOR: light to medium amber, some can be almost transparent

AROMA: cinnamon, cloves, vanilla cupcakes, anise

TASTE: butter, caramel, anise

PAIRS WELL WITH: almost anything you would eat in autumn and at Thanksgiving, such as turkey, stuffing, root vegetables

TASMANIAN LEATHERWOOD

Native to the island state of Tasmania, which is off the coast of Australia. The honey has high vitamin B content and crystallizes very quickly.

COLOR: ochre yellow to light brown to deep reddish amber

AROMA: woody, floral, spicy, pine forest, grape juice

TASTE: woody, intensely floral, spicy, leather, menthol, anise, musky, camphor, peppery

PAIRS WELL WITH: bread, waffles, fruit bread, ginger beer, lentils, smoked cheese

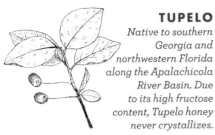

TUPELO

Native to southern Georgia and northwestern Florida along the Apalachicola River Basin. Due to its high fructose content, Tupelo honey never crystallizes.

COLOR: light to medium golden amber with greenish tint

AROMA: stewed fruits, raisins, bread, floral

TASTE: butter, caramel, pineapple, bergamot, toasty, butterscotch, nutmeg, jasmine, pears

PAIRS WELL WITH: biscuits, pie crust, fruit, barbeque

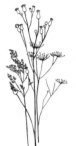

WILDFLOWER

Produced worldwide and popularly used as a base for infusions.

COLOR: variety of hues from blond to auburn, can be dark amber

AROMA: floral, menthol

TASTE: floral, jasmine, prune

PAIRS WELL WITH: stuffed pork loin, Moroccan food, fruit, stuffed chicken, duck, base sauces, breads, cookies, nuts

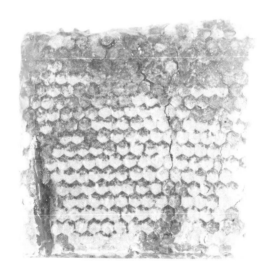

the asheville bee charmer cookbook

A NOTE ON INGREDIENTS

The Asheville Bee Charmer attracts people from many different backgrounds, so it was important to me that the recipes in this book reflect that spirit by being accessible to all kinds of home cooks. You'll notice that there are multiple recipes for each kind of honey (for a full index, see page 198), so you know that if you buy a special jar of delicious artisanal honey, you'll be able to use it in multiple ways in the kitchen. Likewise, many of my recipes use my favorite ingredients—all of which are readily available at the grocery store—over and over again. Here are the most common ones you'll see:

Grapeseed oil. I love using grapeseed oil as a neutral-flavored oil for a number of reasons: it is a relatively "healthy" oil, as it has some monounsaturated fat plus a high level of polyunsaturated fats like omega-6 and omega-9 fatty acids; when used in moderation, grapeseed oil can lower cholesterol levels; it has a moderately high smoke point; it is a non-GMO product; and it is an abundant by-product of winemaking. Terroir plays an important role with grapeseed oil, so make sure you taste a variety of brands before finding the one that you like the most.

Olive oil. Olive oil is a "healthy" oil, as it is a monounsaturated fat. It has a lower smoke point than grapeseed oil, but I still like to use it for cooking certain foods. In general, I use it with Mediterranean-inspired dishes, sauces, and dressings. Depending on the type of olive oil you use, it can have a relatively neutral taste, or it can have a very strong taste that can overpower your food. Terroir plays a really important role with olive oil, not only in terms of color and aroma but also, most importantly, in terms of taste. I prefer to use extra-virgin olive oil because it is lighter and is made from the first pressing of the olives, which doesn't allow high heat or chemicals. After this first pressing, no additional processing or refining occurs. Make sure to taste a variety of oils from different regions and choose the kind that you like the most.

Tamari. This is similar to soy sauce, as it is also made from soybeans. However, it contains little to no wheat. It is darker in color, richer in flavor, and less salty than regular soy sauce. I like to use it because of its balanced flavor and because it is readily available in a gluten-free variety.

Sambal oelek. This is a type of Southeast Asian hot sauce made from hot red chiles, vinegar, and salt. Some varieties may contain garlic, onion, or sugar, but I prefer the plain chili paste. I like to use it because it adds heat to a dish without impacting its flavor. You can usually find it near other Asian ingredients, such as soy sauce.

Aleppo pepper flakes. Aleppo pepper is a variety of hot pepper named for the city of Aleppo, which lies along the Silk Road in northern Syria. Aleppo pepper tastes almost like an ancho chile, but it is oilier and slightly salty. It is dried, deseeded, and then crushed or ground, which is how you usually buy it. I often use it instead of regular red pepper flakes because it has a moderate heat level, some fruity notes, and a hint of cumin flavor. I find it to be much more flavorful than standard red pepper flakes.

TIPS FOR COOKING WITH HONEY

Honey tastes sweeter than granulated sugar. When substituting honey for granulated sugar, you will typically use ¾ cup honey for every 1 cup of granulated sugar. However, depending on the fructose-to-glucose ratio in the honey, some honeys will be sweeter than others. Always taste your honey before using it. If it's really sweet, then use slightly less.

When substituting honey for brown sugar, you will use a little less than ¾ cup honey for every 1 cup of brown sugar, since brown sugar is not as sweet as granulated sugar.

When substituting honey in a baking recipe, you cannot just make a straight substitution. You will have to add more dry ingredients to compensate for the additional moisture. This is less of an issue with a savory recipe, but is still something to keep in mind.

Honey crystallization—when honey turns from a liquid to a semi-solid made up of granules—is a naturally occurring process. This can happen after you open the jar of honey or if it gets cold. If your honey crystallizes, simply put the jar or bottle of honey in some warm water until it melts back into its liquid form.

DIETARY RESTRICTIONS

I have spent much of my culinary career developing recipes for those who follow certain diets, such as gluten free, dairy free, or vegetarian. This kind of cooking comes naturally to me, and when I realized how many of the recipes I developed for this book happened to fall into those categories, I decided to mark them for those of you who may follow those diets. Look out for these icons as you peruse the book. I've also included a comprehensive table that organizes the recipes by dietary restriction in Appendix B (see page 193).

DIET ICONS IN RECIPES

DF	DAIRY FREE
GF	GLUTEN FREE
V	VEGETARIAN

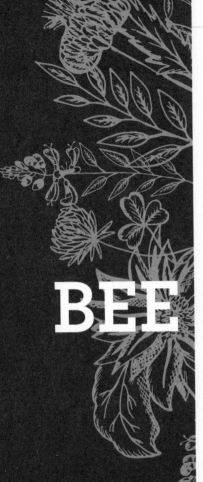

BEE Awake

CHAPTER 1

Breakfast Foods

EVERYDAY GRANOLA

Granola is great as cereal, as a crunchy topping for yogurt, ice cream, or fruit crumble, or just as a snack. Most packaged granola has a lot of sugar in it. This granola recipe is full of flavor but isn't overly sweet. If there are other nuts or dried fruits you prefer, substitute away. The spices work well with a wide variety of fruits and nuts. Since the granola stores well, it's worth it to make a double batch. You can also use this granola as a base for a trail mix with other nuts and some M&M's. ❧ **MAKES 6 CUPS**

3½ cups gluten-free rolled oats (not quick cooking)

½ cup dried, unsweetened cranberries

½ cup raisins

½ cup unsalted, roasted pumpkin seeds

½ cup unsalted, roasted pecans, roughly chopped

½ cup dried apricots, chopped into ¼-inch cubes

1 teaspoon ground cinnamon

1 teaspoon ground ginger

1 teaspoon ground allspice

½ teaspoon ground nutmeg

½ teaspoon kosher salt

¾ cup Corsican blossom honey

1½ teaspoons pure vanilla extract

½ cup unsweetened applesauce

Preheat the oven to 325°F. Line a baking sheet with parchment paper and set it aside.

In a large bowl, mix together the oats, dried cranberries, raisins, pumpkin seeds, pecans, dried apricots, cinnamon, ginger, allspice, nutmeg, and salt. Stir well.

In a small bowl, whisk together the honey, vanilla, and applesauce. Pour the honey mixture over the oat mixture and stir until evenly coated. Spread the granola on the prepared baking sheet.

Bake for 20 minutes, remove the granola from the oven and give it a good stir, then return it to the oven and bake for another 20 minutes, or until golden brown. Remove the granola from the oven and let it cool completely on the baking sheet. The mixture will feel a little damp when you take it out of the oven, but it will dry out as it cools. Store leftover granola in an airtight container at room temperature for up to 2 weeks.

LENTIL BREAKFAST MUFFINS

There are two types of breakfast people: sweet and savory. I am definitely a savory person. I also really like food that is individually portioned. A few years ago I was asked to use lentils in a non-traditional way, and I was intrigued by the idea of creating a high-protein, savory breakfast muffin. As the muffins bake, the lentils almost melt, so you're left with a slightly nutty and smoky flavor. These are a great grab-and-go breakfast option. When I make a batch, depending on how many people are around, I freeze up to a dozen and then take them out as I need them for breakfast. ❧ **MAKES 15 TO 16 MUFFINS**

¾ cup all-purpose flour

½ cup lentil flour

1 teaspoon baking powder

½ teaspoon kosher salt

1½ sticks (¾ cup) unsalted butter, at room temperature

¼ cup firmly packed light brown sugar

¼ cup Tasmanian leatherwood honey

5 large eggs

10 slices cooked bacon, chopped

1 bunch green onions, roughly chopped (1 cup)

1 cup cooked brown lentils

Preheat the oven to 350°F. Grease two standard-sized muffin pans with nonstick cooking spray and set them aside.

In a small bowl, mix together the all-purpose and lentil flours, baking powder, and salt.

In the bowl of a stand mixer fitted with the paddle attachment, cream the butter, brown sugar, and honey on medium speed until light and fluffy, about 5 minutes. Alternate between adding the flour mixture and the eggs to the creamed butter mixture (add the flour mixture in three stages and the eggs in two stages, beginning and ending with the flour). Turn off the mixer, remove the paddle, and fold in the bacon, green onions, and lentils.

Scoop the batter into the prepared muffin pans, filling each cup about three-quarters full. Bake for 25 to 30 minutes, or until the muffins are firm to the touch and cooked through. To check for doneness, insert a toothpick into the center of the muffins. If it comes out clean, they are finished baking.

Remove the muffins from the oven and serve them right away or let them cool to room temperature on a wire rack. Store leftover muffins in an airtight container at room temperature for up to 4 days or in the freezer for up to 6 months.

NOTE *You can typically find lentil flour in an Asian or Indian grocery store. You can also make your own by very finely grinding brown lentils in your blender. Make sure to do a little at a time so that the lentils get finely ground. The texture should feel as fine as all-purpose flour; you don't want to see any chunks of raw lentils.*

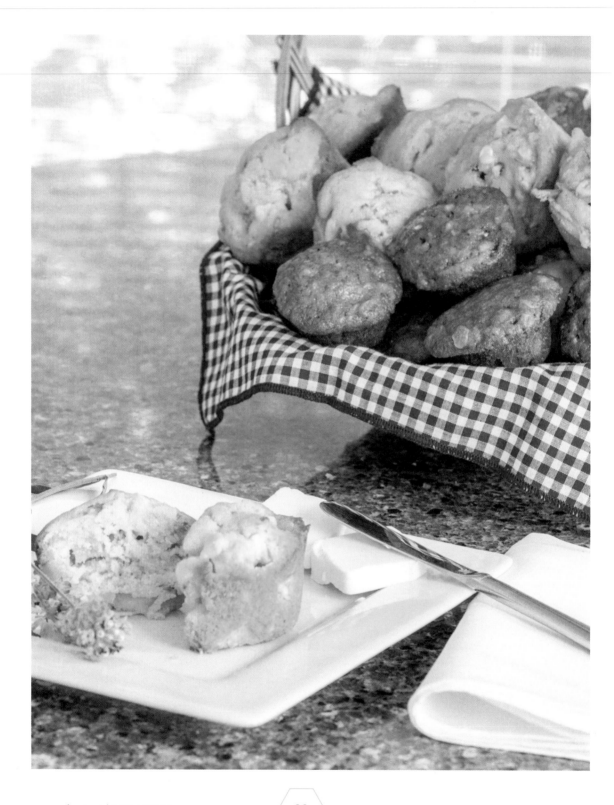

APPLE LAVENDER MUFFINS

Every time I smell lavender, I am always transported to the South of France. I have a couple of lavender plants in my garden, and anytime they flower, I use the flowers, which I dry on a baking sheet for a couple of days, to bake these muffins. The lavender and apple taste great together, and the addition of lavender honey enhances both the natural sweetness of the apple and the fragrant taste of the lavender. These are also fun as an afternoon pick-me-up with a cup of tea. ❧ **MAKES 12 MUFFINS**

1 cup all-purpose flour

½ cup whole wheat flour

2 tablespoons firmly packed light brown sugar

2 teaspoons baking powder

½ teaspoon kosher salt

¼ cup 2% milk

¼ cup lavender honey

2 tablespoons dried lavender flowers

1 stick (½ cup) unsalted butter, melted and cooled slightly

1 large egg, lightly beaten

2 medium Braeburn apples, peeled and cut into ¼-inch cubes (2½ cups)

Unsalted butter and lavender honey, for serving

Preheat the oven to 375°F. Grease a standard-sized muffin pan with nonstick cooking spray and set it aside.

In a large bowl, whisk together the all-purpose and whole wheat flours, brown sugar, baking powder, and salt. Add the milk, honey, lavender, butter, and egg. With a rubber spatula, stir until just combined. Fold in the apples.

Spoon the mixture into the prepared muffin pan, filling each cup about three-quarters full. Bake for 25 to 30 minutes, or until the muffins are golden brown and cooked through. To check for doneness, insert a toothpick into the center of the muffins. If it comes out clean, they are finished baking.

Remove the muffins from the oven and let them cool for 5 minutes in the pan, then transfer them to a wire rack to cool completely. Serve with some butter and additional lavender honey. Store leftover muffins in an airtight container at room temperature for up to 4 days or in the freezer for up to 6 months.

Pictured at left, from top: Carrot Orange Sunflower Date Muffins (p. 33); Zucchini Carrot Nut Mini Muffins (p. 35); Apple Lavender Muffins

FRENCH TOAST WITH BERRY COULIS

What to do with leftover challah or brioche? The best way I can think to use it up is to make French toast. There is nothing better than rich, custard-soaked bread sautéed in butter, served with a fresh coulis, and sprinkled with some powdered sugar. It's rich and satisfying, and it will transport you to France in no time. This also makes a great late-night snack! ❧ **MAKES 4 SERVINGS**

4 large eggs, beaten
1 cup half-and-half
½ teaspoon kosher salt
1 teaspoon freshly grated lemon zest

8 slices brioche or challah bread, preferably 1 day old
1 stick (½ cup) unsalted butter
Powdered sugar, for garnish
1–2 cups Berry Coulis (page 176), for serving

Place a griddle or sauté pan over medium-high heat until it's hot but not smoking.

In a small bowl, whisk together the eggs, half-and-half, salt, and lemon zest. Pour the mixture into a shallow baking dish. Place the bread slices in the egg mixture and soak them for 1 to 2 minutes. Flip the bread slices and soak them on the other side for another 1 to 2 minutes.

Melt the butter on the hot griddle or sauté pan. Cook the bread for 3 to 4 minutes per side, or until golden brown.

Place two slices of the bread on each of four plates. Dust with the powdered sugar. Add ¼ to ½ cup of the Berry Coulis to each plate and serve.

CARROT ORANGE SUNFLOWER DATE MUFFINS

These muffins, despite being a healthy alternative to a traditional sweet muffin, are full of flavor and natural sweetness. They are dense and provide great energy when you are on the go and need a quick breakfast. These are also great with dried cranberries or cherries as a substitute for the dates. ✤ **MAKES 18 MUFFINS**

1½ cups all-purpose flour

1½ cups whole wheat flour

1 cup gluten-free rolled oats (not quick cooking)

½ cup firmly packed light brown sugar

½ cup unsalted, roasted sunflower seeds

½ cup dates, pitted and cut into ¼-inch cubes

1 tablespoon + 1 teaspoon baking powder

½ teaspoon ground cinnamon

1 teaspoon ground ginger

1½ cups grated carrot

¼ cup carrot honey

¼ cup orange blossom honey

1½ cups freshly squeezed orange juice

¼ cup unsweetened applesauce

2 tablespoons grapeseed oil

Preheat the oven to 350°F. Grease two standard-sized muffin pans with nonstick cooking spray and set them aside.

In a large bowl, whisk together the all-purpose and whole wheat flours, oats, brown sugar, sunflower seeds, dates, baking powder, cinnamon, and ginger. Add the carrot, carrot and orange blossom honeys, orange juice, applesauce, and oil. With a rubber spatula, stir until just combined. Spoon the mixture into the prepared muffin pans, filling each cup about three-quarters full.

Bake for 30 minutes, or until the muffins are golden brown and cooked through. To check for doneness, insert a toothpick into the center of the muffins. If it comes out clean, they are finished baking.

Remove the muffins from the oven and let them cool for 5 minutes in the pan, then transfer them to a wire rack to cool completely. Serve at room temperature. Store leftover muffins in an airtight container in the refrigerator for up to 7 days or in the freezer for up to 6 months.

Pictured on p. 30

AMARANTH, NUT, AND SEED BARS

These gluten-free bars are super easy to make and great to take on the go, whether you are hiking, running, or just going to the playground with your kids. Amaranth is good as a plain seed, but it's even better when it's popped. It takes on a slightly nutty, crunchy quality. Just be careful when you're popping the amaranth because it will fly around! 🐝 **MAKES 8 BARS**

1 cup amaranth

½ cup salted, roasted sunflower seeds

½ cup salted, roasted pumpkin seeds

½ cup unsalted, roasted almonds, roughly chopped

¾ cup fir honey

6 tablespoons unsalted butter

Grease an 8 × 8-inch baking pan with nonstick cooking spray and set it aside.

Place a small, high-sided saucepan over high heat. Place 1 tablespoon of the amaranth in the bottom of the pan, shaking it constantly until the amaranth pops, about 20 to 25 seconds. Make sure not to let the seeds burn. They will look like tiny popped popcorn kernels. Place the popped amaranth in a medium bowl. Repeat this process for the rest of the amaranth. Add the sunflower seeds, pumpkin seeds, and almonds to the popped amaranth and stir well.

In a medium saucepan over medium-high heat, combine the honey and butter. Let the mixture heat up for about 7 minutes, stirring occasionally, until it registers 234°F on a high-heat instant-read thermometer. Remove the pan from the heat. Add the amaranth mixture and stir until it's well coated.

Press the mixture into the prepared pan and set it aside to cool completely. If you cooked the honey-butter mixture long enough, the mixture should harden. If it doesn't, you can place the pan in the freezer for about 1 hour and it will harden. To serve, cut into eight (2 × 4-inch) bars. Store leftover bars in an airtight container in the refrigerator for up to 1 week (if they last that long!).

Pictured on p. 52

ZUCCHINI CARROT NUT MINI MUFFINS

To mix things up a bit, I make these muffins in a mini version. I wouldn't call these super healthy, but they are on the healthy side, since the recipe incorporates whole wheat flour and oats, which are high in fiber and other essential nutrients. With lots of spices and loads of carrot and zucchini, these really pack a taste punch. If you don't have a mini muffin pan, make them in a regular-sized muffin pan instead. ❧ **MAKES 54 TO 56 MINI MUFFINS**

1 cup all-purpose flour

1 cup whole wheat flour

½ cup gluten-free rolled oats (not quick cooking)

1 cup firmly packed light brown sugar

1 teaspoon kosher salt

2 teaspoons baking powder

1 teaspoon baking soda

1 teaspoon ground cinnamon

½ teaspoon ground nutmeg

1 teaspoon ground ginger

½ cup walnuts, roughly chopped

1 cup grated carrot

1 cup grated zucchini

4 large eggs, lightly beaten

½ cup grapeseed oil

½ cup sourwood honey

¼ cup unsweetened applesauce

Preheat the oven to 350°F. Grease three mini muffin pans with nonstick cooking spray and set them aside.

In a large bowl, whisk together the all-purpose and whole wheat flours, oats, brown sugar, salt, baking powder, baking soda, cinnamon, nutmeg, ginger, and walnuts. Add the carrot, zucchini, eggs, oil, honey, and applesauce. Mix well with a rubber spatula. Spoon the mixture into the prepared muffin pans, filling each cup about three-quarters full.

Bake for 25 minutes, or until the muffins are golden brown and cooked through. To check for doneness, insert a toothpick into the center of the muffins. If it comes out clean, they are finished baking.

Remove the muffins from the oven and let them cool for 5 minutes in the pans, then transfer them to a wire rack to cool completely. Serve the muffins at room temperature. Store leftover muffins in an airtight container at room temperature for up to 4 days or in the freezer for up to 6 months.

Pictured on p. 30

LEMON RICOTTA BLUEBERRY PANCAKES

Adding ricotta to pancake batter gives you a super fluffy pancake with an almost creamy texture. Throw in some fresh lemon zest and blueberries and you have a rich, delicious breakfast treat. I always make a big batch of pancakes and refrigerate or freeze the leftover cooked ones. That way, I can have great pancakes in a flash, any time I want. ❧ **MAKES 4 SERVINGS**

2 cups all-purpose flour
1 teaspoon baking powder
½ teaspoon baking soda
½ teaspoon kosher salt
2 tablespoons acacia honey
1½ cups whole milk ricotta

2 large eggs
1½ cups buttermilk
Zest of 1 large lemon
½ teaspoon pure vanilla extract
3½ cups fresh blueberries, divided
¼–½ cup blueberry honey

Place a griddle over medium heat (it will take about 5 to 7 minutes to reach the right temperature). Preheat the oven to 150°F or 200°F.

In a large bowl, whisk together the flour, baking powder, baking soda, and salt. In a medium bowl, whisk together the acacia honey, ricotta, eggs, buttermilk, lemon zest, and vanilla. Pour the ricotta mixture into the bowl with the flour mixture. Mix well with a large spoon until the ingredients are just incorporated. Set aside.

Once the griddle is hot and just beginning to smoke, grease it with nonstick cooking spray. Pour ¼ cup of the batter onto the griddle for each pancake. Place about 12 of the blueberries on each pancake. Cook for 3 to 4 minutes, or until you see bubbles on the top and the bottom is lightly browned. Gently flip the pancakes (you don't want to smash the blueberries) and cook for another 3 to 4 minutes, or until they are cooked through and lightly spring back to the touch. Repeat this process until you have used all of the batter. Reserve the extra blueberries (you should have about 1 cup left) for the garnish. To keep the freshly made pancakes warm, place them on a platter in the oven as you continue to make the rest.

To serve, place two or three pancakes on each of four plates. Top each serving with 1 to 2 tablespoons of the blueberry honey and garnish with ¼ cup of the remaining blueberries. Serve immediately. Store leftover pancakes in an airtight container in the refrigerator for up to 4 days or in the freezer for up to 3 months.

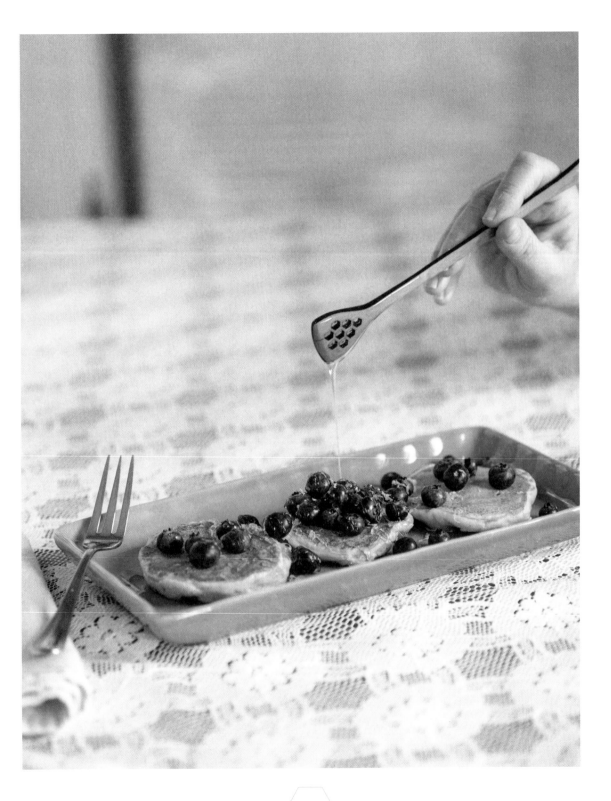

the asheville bee charmer cookbook

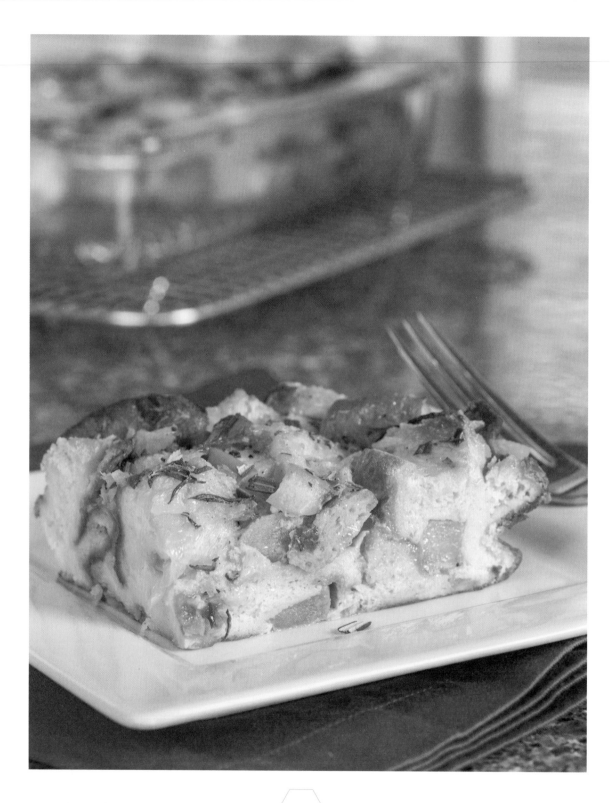

BREAKFAST BREAD PUDDING

The second best way to use up leftover challah or brioche is a bread pudding. This bread pudding is both sweet and savory. The apples and honey add sweetness that balances the chicken sausage, sharp cheddar, and rich, buttery bread. This is a great casserole to make on a Sunday and enjoy as leftovers (if there are any) during the week! ❧ **MAKES 8 TO 10 SERVINGS**

2 tablespoons grapeseed oil, divided

1 (12-ounce) package apple- or sage-flavored chicken sausage, cut on the bias into ½-inch-thick slices

1 large yellow onion, cut into ¼-inch cubes (about 2 cups)

1 large Braeburn apple, cored and cut into ¼-inch cubes (about 1½ cups)

1 teaspoon kosher salt

½ teaspoon freshly ground black pepper

2 tablespoons Asheville Bee Charmer's Rosemary-Infused Honey

2 tablespoons sage honey

1 (15-ounce) loaf brioche or challah bread, cut into 1-inch cubes

4 ounces sharp cheddar, grated

1 tablespoon minced fresh rosemary

8 large eggs

1½ cups whole or 2% milk

Preheat the oven to 350°F. Grease a 9 × 13-inch baking dish with nonstick cooking spray and set it aside.

In a large sauté pan, warm 1 tablespoon of the grapeseed oil over medium-high heat, until it's hot but not smoking. Add the sausage and sauté until the slices are nicely browned on both sides, about 3 to 5 minutes. Transfer the sausage to a medium bowl and set it aside.

In the same sauté pan, warm the remaining tablespoon of grapeseed oil over medium-high heat. Add the onion, apple, salt, and pepper and sauté until the onion and apple are soft and slightly browned, about 5 to 8 minutes. Remove the apple-onion mixture from the heat and add it to the bowl with the sausage. Add the Rosemary-Infused Honey and sage honey, toss, and set aside.

Place the bread in the prepared baking dish in an even layer. Sprinkle with the cheddar. Pour the sausage mixture over top and gently stir until everything is well incorporated. Sprinkle with the rosemary.

In the same bowl you used for the sausage mixture, whisk together the eggs and milk until well emulsified. Pour this mixture over the bread. Press gently so that all the bread can absorb the egg mixture and it is evenly incorporated.

Let the bread pudding rest for 15 minutes at room temperature, then transfer it to the oven and bake for 1 hour, or until it is lightly browned on top. Serve immediately. Store leftovers in an airtight container in the refrigerator for up to 7 days.

NOTE *If you know you are going to have a busy morning, you can prepare the bread pudding the night before, cover it with plastic wrap, and let it soak overnight in the refrigerator. Make sure you let it come to room temperature before you put it in the oven to bake.*

BEE Appetizing

CHAPTER 2

Small Plates and Snacks

HONEY WHEAT SOFT PRETZEL BITES

Soft pretzels are absolutely delicious, whether eaten plain or dipped in cheese sauce, marinara sauce, or honey mustard. Many soft pretzels are really big, and a lot of times I just want part of one—not the whole thing. Rather than letting pretzels go stale, why not make them bite sized? You can have as many or as few as you want. And if you make a big batch, you can freeze them after they are baked and cooled. Reheat them in the oven or a toaster oven for a great anytime snack. 🐝 **MAKES 12 SERVINGS**

1½ cups warm water (about 100°F)
1 tablespoon fir honey
4½ teaspoons active dry yeast
2 teaspoons kosher salt
3½ cups whole wheat flour

¼ cup baking soda
1 cup hot water (about 160°F)
6 tablespoons melted Honey Butter (page 177)
Sesame seeds and/or kosher salt, for topping
Honey Mustard (page 174), for serving

In the bowl of a stand mixer fitted with a dough hook, whisk together the warm water, honey, and yeast. Let the mixture stand for about 5 minutes, or until the yeast starts to foam.

Add the salt and flour to the bowl. Mix the ingredients with the dough hook on low speed until just incorporated. Increase the speed to medium and mix for 5 minutes, or until the dough is smooth and elastic. Place the dough in a lightly oiled bowl. Cover with plastic wrap and let the dough rise for 1 hour, or until it has doubled in size.

Preheat the oven to 475°F. Line two baking sheets with parchment paper and set them aside.

In a shallow bowl or container, dissolve the baking soda in the hot water.

Turn the pretzel dough out onto a lightly floured, clean work surface. Divide the dough into 12 equal pieces. Roll each piece so that it looks like a piece of rope and is about ½ inch thick. Using a sharp knife, cut each rope into 1-inch pieces.

Dip each piece of dough into the baking soda bath and place them about ½ inch apart on the prepared baking sheets. Brush each pretzel with the melted Honey Butter. Sprinkle with sesame seeds, kosher salt, or both.

Bake for 5 to 6 minutes, or until the pretzels are nicely browned. Remove them from the oven and let them cool slightly. Serve warm with the Honey Mustard. Store leftover pretzels in an airtight container at room temperature for 1 to 2 days or in the freezer for up to 6 months.

NOTE *To make sweet pretzels, brush the pretzels with melted Honey Butter made with chai honey, and sprinkle them with cinnamon sugar instead of the sesame seeds or salt.*

HONEY WHOLE WHEAT PIZZA CRUST

Homemade pizza is one of the tastiest and simplest things to make. It's great for a family meal, at a party, or even as a snack. You can customize your pizza so easily using marinara sauce, pesto sauce, white sauce, or just olive oil on the crust. Top with anything you like, from cooked meat or poultry to fresh or cooked veggies, fruit, nuts, and/or your choice of cheese. Be creative! ✻ **MAKES 6 INDIVIDUAL PIZZA CRUSTS**

2¼ teaspoons active dry yeast

1 cup warm water (about 100°F)

1 tablespoon wildflower honey

1½ cups whole wheat flour

1 cup all-purpose flour

1½ teaspoons kosher salt

2 tablespoons olive oil

Up to ½ cup cornmeal, for dusting the dough

In the bowl of a stand mixer fitted with the dough hook, whisk together the yeast, warm water, and honey. Let the mixture stand for about 5 minutes, or until the yeast starts to foam.

Add the whole wheat flour, all-purpose flour, salt, and olive oil to the bowl. Mix the dough on low speed until the flour has been incorporated. Increase the speed to medium and mix until the dough comes together into a ball, about 5 minutes. You want the dough to be smooth and elastic (if you poke your finger into the dough, it should spring back). If the dough looks crumbly, add more lukewarm water, 1 tablespoon at a time. If the dough looks too wet, add more all-purpose flour, 1 tablespoon at a time.

Cover the dough with plastic wrap and let it rise at room temperature for 1 hour, or until it has doubled in size.

Preheat the oven to 450°F. Line two baking sheets with parchment paper and set them aside.

Punch down the dough, then divide it into six equal balls. Sprinkle a little cornmeal on a clean work surface. Roll out each dough ball until it is about ¼ inch thick. Fold the edges of the dough inward to form a crust. Use a fork to gently prick holes all over the dough.

Place the crusts on the prepared baking sheets. Bake for 7 to 8 minutes, or until the crusts are lightly browned. Remove them from the oven and let them cool for about 5 minutes, then top with whatever sauce or ingredients you want.

NOTE *If you don't want to use all the pizza dough at once, wrap the uncooked individual balls with plastic wrap and place them in a freezer-proof baggie. They will keep in the freezer for up to 3 months. When you want to use them, thaw them in the refrigerator and then roll them out.*

To make a pizza with your dough, once you have par-baked the crust, top each crust with ¼ to ½ cup of your favorite sauce. Then place any toppings you might like on the pizza, including your favorite cheese. Bake your pizza for another 6 to 7 minutes in a 450°F oven, or until your toppings are nicely browned and the cheese is bubbly.

BRIE, CRANBERRY, AND ALMOND PHYLLO CUPS

Hands down, these have to be the easiest appetizers you will ever make. From start to finish, they only take about 15 minutes. I used to make these with raspberry jam, but one Thanksgiving I had some leftover cranberry orange sauce and thought, why not? I have never gone back to raspberry jam. There's something about the sweet and tangy cranberry sauce that adds depth to the Brie and ensures this to be an appetizer your friends and family are sure to ask you to make again and again. ❧ **MAKES 45 PHYLLO CUPS**

45 mini pre-baked phyllo cups
8 ounces Brie, with rind removed
About ½ cup Cranberry Orange Sauce (page 174)

About ¼ cup cranberry honey
About ½ cup sliced almonds

Preheat the oven to 350°F. Line a baking sheet with parchment paper, and set the phyllo cups on top.

Cut the Brie into ½-inch cubes. Place 1 cube in each phyllo cup. Add ½ teaspoon of the Cranberry Orange Sauce on top of each piece of Brie. Then add ¼ teaspoon of the cranberry honey on top of the cranberry sauce. Finish each cup by placing ½ teaspoon of the sliced almonds on top of the honey.

Bake for 8 to 10 minutes, or until the cheese is just melted. Remove the cups from the oven and serve them immediately, or let them cool and serve them at room temperature. The phyllo cups will soften the longer they sit. Store leftover cups in an airtight container in the refrigerator for 1 to 2 days.

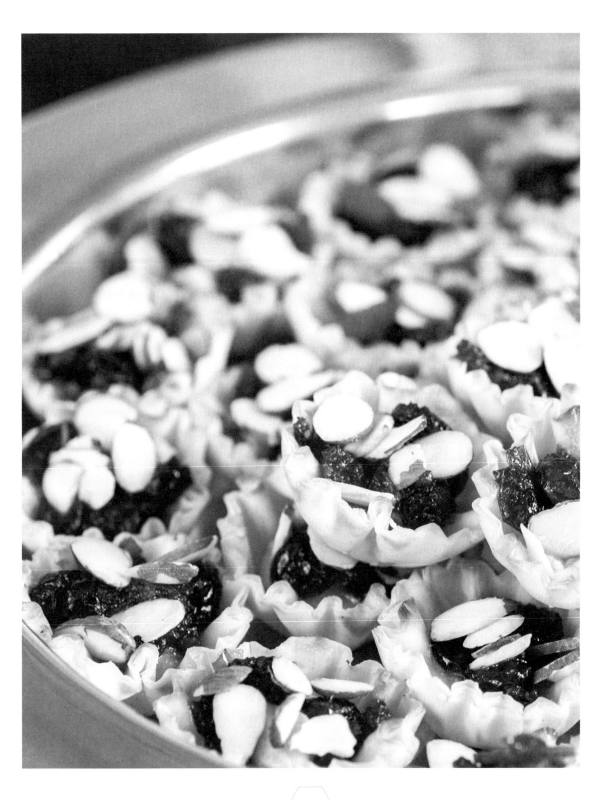

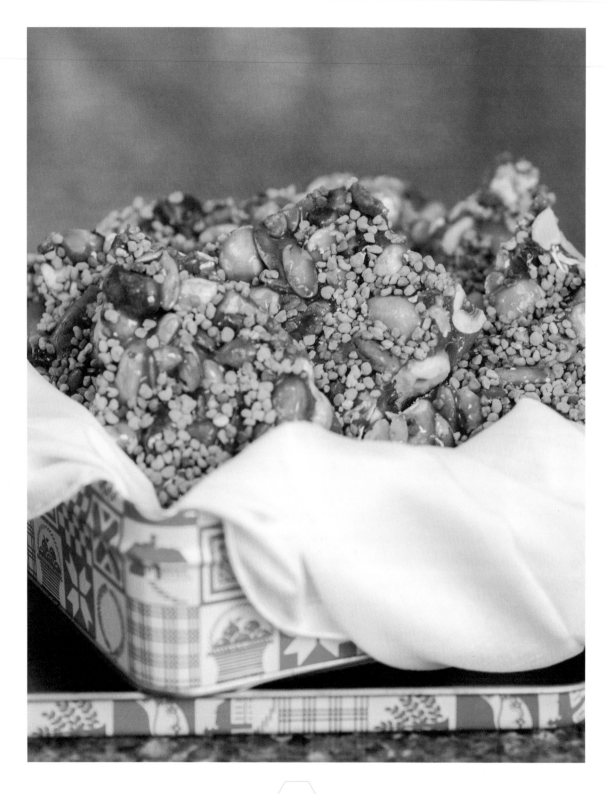

BEE POLLEN NUT BRITTLE

When I started thinking about recipes for this book, I knew I wanted to make a nut brittle that used honey in the base. I chose fir honey for this recipe because of the rich caramel flavor it adds to the end product. This brittle is packed to the gills with nuts—can there ever be too many nuts? But the most special ingredient is the bee pollen that's sprinkled on top. It adds a depth and richness of flavor that is unforgettable. When I make it, I hide some, because it is gone before you know it! 🐝 MAKES 1 BAKING SHEET OF BRITTLE

¾ cup fir honey

¾ cup raw cane sugar

¼ cup unsalted butter

½ cup water

½ teaspoon baking soda

½ teaspoon pure vanilla extract

½ cup salted, roasted cashews

½ cup roasted, shelled pistachios

½ cup roasted, halved pecans

½ cup salted, roasted peanuts

½ cup salted, roasted pumpkin seeds

½ cup roasted hazelnuts

½ cup bee pollen

Line a baking sheet with parchment paper and set it aside.

In a medium saucepan over medium-high heat, combine the honey, sugar, butter, and water and cook for 10 to 15 minutes, stirring occasionally, until the caramel is golden brown and registers 300°F on a high-heat instant-read thermometer.

Remove the pan from the heat and carefully add the baking soda (watch out as it will foam); stir until the baking soda is completely incorporated. Add the vanilla, cashews, pistachios, pecans, peanuts, pumpkin seeds, and hazelnuts. Stir to coat well.

Pour the brittle mixture onto the prepared baking sheet, and spread it in a thin layer using a heatproof nonstick spatula. Sprinkle the bee pollen on top.

Set the brittle aside at room temperature for about 45 minutes, until completely cool and firmly set. Break the brittle apart. Store the brittle in an airtight container at room temperature for up to 2 weeks or in the freezer for up to 6 months.

ROASTED PEAR, BLUE CHEESE, AND WALNUT PHYLLO BITES

This appetizer is similar to spanakopita, but instead of spinach, you fill the phyllo with roasted pear, crumbled blue cheese, and chopped walnuts—one of my favorite flavor combinations. It reminds me of tasting wine in northern California in the fall. The secret ingredient is a dab of lavender honey, which enhances all the other flavors. **MAKES 25 PHYLLO TRIANGLES**

3 ripe but firm Bosc or Anjou pears, peeled, cored, and cut into ¼-inch cubes

2 tablespoons olive oil

½ teaspoon kosher salt

¼ teaspoon freshly ground black pepper

1 stick (½ cup) unsalted butter, melted

1 (16-ounce) package phyllo dough (14 × 18-inch sheets), thawed in the refrigerator

4 ounces blue cheese, crumbled

½ cup unsalted, roasted walnuts, roughly chopped

2½ tablespoons lavender honey

Preheat the oven to 450°F. Line a baking sheet with parchment paper and set it aside.

In a small bowl, combine the pears, olive oil, salt, and pepper. Toss well to make sure the pears are evenly coated.

Put the pears on the prepared baking sheet and roast for 25 minutes, or until they are browned. Remove the pears from the oven and set them aside. Reduce the oven temperature to 400°F. Line another baking sheet with parchment paper and set it aside.

To assemble the triangles, take one piece of phyllo and brush it with butter. Lay another sheet of phyllo on top and brush with butter. Place a third piece of phyllo on top and brush with butter. Using a pizza cutter, slice the layered phyllo sheets horizontally into five equal-size strips.

Place 1 tablespoon of the roasted pears on one end of each of the five strips. Add 1 teaspoon of the blue cheese, 1 teaspoon of the walnuts, and ¼ teaspoon of the lavender honey to the pears. Fold each phyllo strip in a triangle, like a flag. Brush each triangle with melted butter and place it on the prepared baking sheet.

Repeat this process until all the filling has been used.

Bake the phyllo triangles for 15 minutes, or until they are golden brown. Remove them from the oven and let them cool. The triangles can be served warm or at room temperature. Store leftovers in an airtight container in the refrigerator for up to 4 days.

NOTE *It's easiest to work with phyllo if you keep it cool and moist. You should cover the phyllo with plastic wrap and then a damp towel. If you cover the sheets directly with a damp towel, you will get the phyllo soggy and it will be unusable.*

CHOCOLATE HONEY ALMOND NO-BAKE GRANOLA BARS

A typical granola bar is loaded with sugar, but it is easy to make your own (healthier) bars, especially if you don't have to bake them. Using a combination of oats, crispy brown rice cereal, and almonds provides these bars with a soft yet crunchy texture. Add some chocolate chips and cocoa honey to the mix, and you have a sweet, satisfying, wholesome treat in no time. ❧ MAKES 8 BARS

2 cups gluten-free rolled oats
(not quick cooking)

1 cup crispy brown rice cereal

½ cup unsalted, roasted almonds,
roughly chopped

½ teaspoon kosher salt

¼ cup unsalted butter

⅓ cup Asheville Bee Charmer's
Cocoa-Infused Honey

1 heaping tablespoon dark brown sugar

½ teaspoon pure vanilla extract

½ cup mini semisweet chocolate chips

Grease an 8 × 8-inch pan with nonstick cooking spray and set it aside.

In a large bowl, combine the oats, brown rice cereal, almonds, and salt, and mix well.

In a small saucepan, heat the butter, honey, and brown sugar over medium-high heat until the mixture begins to boil. Reduce the heat to low and cook the mixture until it registers 234°F on a high-heat instant-read thermometer. Remove the pan from the heat and stir in the vanilla.

Pour the honey mixture over the oat mixture and stir until everything is well coated. Carefully stir in the chocolate chips (they will melt a little bit).

Pour the granola into the prepared pan. Place a piece of parchment paper over the granola and press down so that it's evenly and firmly packed. Refrigerate for 1 hour, or until the granola is set.

With a sharp knife, cut the granola into eight (4 × 2-inch) bars. Keep them refrigerated until you're ready to eat. They can be stored in an airtight container in the refrigerator for up to 1 week or in the freezer for up to 6 months.

Pictured on p. 52

HONEY HERB CASHEW HUMMUS

Raw cashews are great as a base for high-protein, healthy-fat vegetarian dips and spreads, making this hummus even more nutrient dense than the regular stuff. This creamy, robust dip pairs great with mixed crudités, pita chips, or your favorite crackers. Throw in some fresh herbs and a touch of honey and you have a real crowd-pleaser. **MAKES ABOUT 2 CUPS**

1½ cups raw cashews

¼ cup tahini

¼ cup olive oil

¼ cup freshly squeezed lemon juice

¼ cup cold water

1 tablespoon Asheville Bee Charmer's Rosemary-Infused Honey

2 large cloves garlic, smashed

¼ cup minced fresh flat-leaf parsley

1 tablespoon minced fresh oregano

1½ tablespoons minced fresh cilantro

1½ tablespoons minced fresh mint

1 green onion, sliced ⅛ inch thick

1 teaspoon kosher salt

Mixed crudités, for serving

Pita chips or crackers, for serving

Place the cashews in a small bowl. Add enough warm water (about 100°F) to cover the nuts and let them soak for 1 hour at room temperature. Drain.

Place the drained cashews in the bowl of a food processor. Pulse them until they are finely chopped. Add the remaining ingredients, except for the crudités and pita chips, and process for 3 to 5 minutes, or until the mixture is smooth. If the mixture still looks chunky, add more water, 1 tablespoon at a time, to get the dip to a smooth consistency.

Serve with mixed crudités, pita chips, or your favorite crackers. Store leftover hummus in an airtight container in the refrigerator for up to 7 days.

LENTIL ENERGY BARS

Cookie bars as a sweet snack have been a favorite in our family since I was a little girl. When I was exploring the use of lentils in nontraditional ways, I wondered if I could use them to modify chocolate chip cookie bars and make them healthier but still taste great; the result are these bars. They are really a cross between a cookie bar and good fruitcake. These provide a great afternoon energy boost from the protein-packed lentils, dried fruits, and pumpkin seeds. The chocolate chips just enhance all the great flavors. **MAKES 15 BARS**

1½ sticks (¾ cup) unsalted butter, at room temperature

½ cup firmly packed dark brown sugar

½ cup buckwheat honey

3 large eggs

1 cup lentil flour

2 cups gluten-free rolled oats (not quick cooking)

1 teaspoon baking soda

1 teaspoon ground cinnamon

½ teaspoon ground cardamom

1 teaspoon kosher salt

2 cups cooked brown lentils

½ cup dates, pitted and cut into ¼-inch cubes

½ cup dried apricots, cut into ¼-inch cubes

½ cup dried cranberries

½ cup salted, roasted pumpkin seeds

¾ cup bittersweet chocolate chips

Preheat the oven to 375°F. Grease a 9 × 13-inch baking pan with nonstick cooking spray and set it aside.

In the bowl of a stand mixer fitted with the paddle attachment, combine the butter, brown sugar, and honey. Mix on medium speed until everything is well incorporated, about 5 minutes. Reduce the speed to low and add the eggs one at a time, making sure each one is fully incorporated before adding the next.

Add the lentil flour, rolled oats, baking soda, cinnamon, cardamom, salt, and lentils. Mix until just combined. Add the dates, apricots, cranberries, pumpkin seeds, and chocolate chips. Mix until just incorporated.

Pour the mixture into the prepared pan. Bake for 25 to 30 minutes, or until golden brown and cooked through. To check for doneness, insert a toothpick into the center of the pan. If it comes out clean, it is cooked through.

Remove the pan from the oven and let it cool thoroughly before cutting into squares. Serve at room temperature. Store leftover bars in an airtight container at room temperature for 4 to 5 days or in the freezer for up to 6 months.

NOTE *You can typically find lentil flour in an Asian or Indian grocery store, but you can also make your own. See page 29 for guidance.*

the asheville bee charmer cookbook

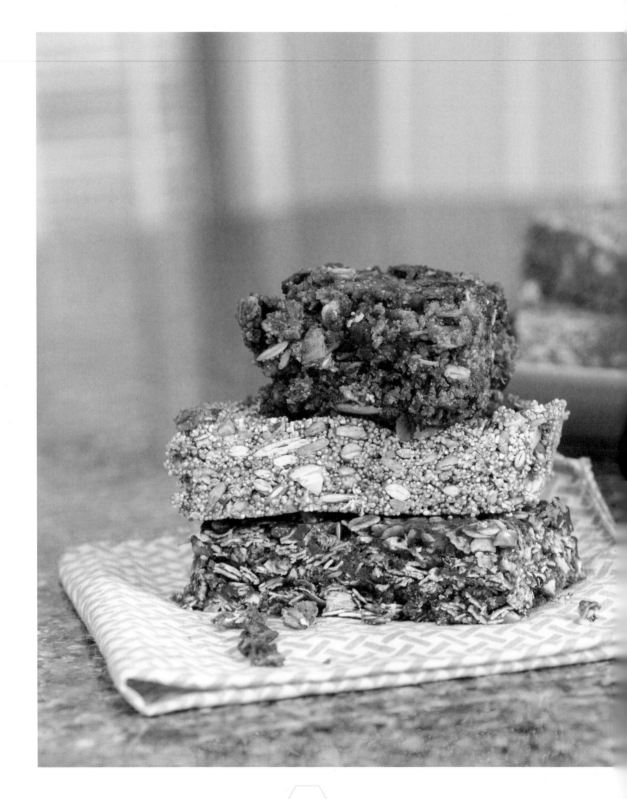

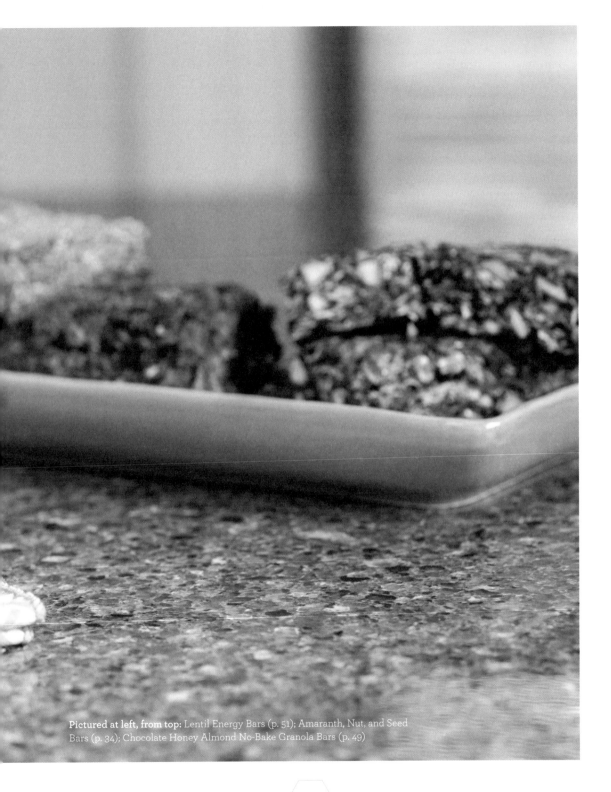

Pictured at left, from top: Lentil Energy Bars (p. 51); Amaranth, Nut, and Seed Bars (p. 34); Chocolate Honey Almond No-Bake Granola Bars (p. 49)

TROPICAL OAT, NUT, AND CHOCOLATE BARS

I first made a version of these bars in culinary school in a nutritional cooking class. They are a cross between a chewy granola bar and a fruit and nut bar. The bars use a mix of four honeys, each contributing a unique flavor profile. The tropical flavors will take you back to your last beach vacation! **MAKES 24 BARS**

1½ cups gluten-free rolled oats (not quick cooking)

½ cup roasted sesame seeds

1½ cups dried apricots, cut into ¼-inch cubes

1½ cups raisins

1 cup unsweetened shredded coconut

1 cup unsalted, roasted peanuts, roughly chopped

1 cup unsalted, roasted almonds, roughly chopped

½ cup almond flour

1½ cups bittersweet chocolate chips

2 tablespoons unsalted butter

¼ cup acacia honey

¼ cup tupelo honey

¼ cup wildflower honey

¼ cup meadowfoam honey

¾ cup firmly packed dark brown sugar

1¼ cups creamy peanut butter

2 tablespoons freshly grated orange zest

Grease a 9 × 13-inch baking pan with nonstick cooking spray and set it aside.

In a large bowl, mix together the oats, sesame seeds, apricots, raisins, coconut, peanuts, almonds, almond flour, and chocolate chips.

In a small saucepan set over medium heat, combine the butter, acacia and tupelo honeys, brown sugar, peanut butter, and zest. Cook, stirring frequently, until the mixture reaches a smooth, pourable consistency, about 5 to 7 minutes. Pour the honey mixture over the oat mixture and stir to combine (the chocolate will melt slightly). Make sure that everything is well coated.

Pour the mixture into the prepared pan. Cover with parchment paper and press firmly. Cover and refrigerate until firm, about 4 hours.

Cut into 24 bars. Store them in an airtight container in the refrigerator until you're ready to eat. These bars will keep for up to 1 week in the refrigerator or 6 months in the freezer.

CANDIED WALNUTS

Candied walnuts are great as a snack, with a glass of wine, sprinkled on a salad, or sprinkled on ice cream. There are lots of ways to make candied nuts, but for me, this is the easiest way. You can also substitute the walnuts with almonds, cashews, peanuts, or pecans. If you want to have a salty candied nut, use a salted nut. Roasting the nuts before candying them will add a richer flavor, but this is totally optional. Whichever nut you choose, just be careful not to let them burn! 🐝 **MAKES 1 CUP**

1 cup walnuts
¼ cup wildflower honey

In a small saucepan over medium-high heat, bring the nuts and honey to a boil. Boil for 3 to 5 minutes, or until the honey thickens and starts to caramelize. Shake the pan every minute or so, to make sure all the nuts are evenly coated and to prevent them from burning. There should be hardly any honey left at the bottom of the pan.

Pour the nuts onto a cooling rack lined with parchment paper. Let them cool completely. Store them in an airtight container at room temperature for up to 2 weeks. Do not store them in the refrigerator. Use the candied nuts on salads or eat them as a snack.

NOTE *To make spicy nuts, you can substitute Asheville Bee Charmer's Firecracker Hot Honey, Smokin' Hot Honey, or Chai-Infused Honey.*

SPICY THAI VEGETABLE EGG ROLLS

Egg rolls are always a great starter for a Thai meal. They also make a tasty afternoon snack when you want something light that's not too filling. It's a great way to eat vegetables! Usually egg rolls are fried, but you can bake them to make a much healthier and less messy version. These egg rolls are pretty spicy. If you want to cut down on the heat, seed and devein the jalapeño. **MAKES 8 TO 10 EGG ROLLS**

2 tablespoons tamari

1 tablespoon freshly squeezed lime juice

1 tablespoon ginger-infused honey

1 tablespoon Asheville Bee Charmer's Firecracker Hot Honey

2 tablespoons rice wine vinegar

2 tablespoons grapeseed oil

3 cloves garlic, minced

1 jalapeño, minced (including the seeds)

½ medium green bell pepper, seeded and cut into ¼-inch pieces (½ cup)

½ medium red bell pepper, seeded and cut into ¼-inch pieces (½ cup)

6 shiitake mushrooms, stemmed and cut into ¼-inch pieces

6 medium leaves Napa cabbage, shredded (3 cups)

3 green onions, minced

1 tablespoon minced fresh ginger

1 (16-ounce) package egg roll wrappers

Sweet and Sour Sauce (page 179), for serving

In a small bowl, whisk together the tamari, lime juice, honeys, and vinegar. Set aside.

In a large sauté pan set over medium-high heat, heat the oil until it's hot but not yet smoking. Add the garlic and jalapeño and cook for about 1 minute. Add the green and red bell peppers and cook for 2 minutes. Add the mushrooms and cook for 2 minutes, or until the mushrooms have softened. Add the cabbage and cook until it wilts, about 2 minutes. Add the green onions and ginger and cook for 1 minute. Add the reserved tamari mixture and cook until it has evaporated, about 2 minutes. Remove the pan from the heat.

Preheat the oven to 425°F. Line a baking sheet with parchment paper and grease it with nonstick cooking spray.

Place an egg roll wrapper on a clean, dry surface. Wipe some water along the edges of the wrapper. Spoon about 2 to 3 tablespoons of the filling along one side of the wrapper, leaving an approximately 1-inch border on each side. Fold the bottom of the wrapper over the filling and then fold in the sides. Roll up the egg roll; it will look like a little burrito. Place the egg roll seam-side down on the prepared baking sheet. Repeat this process until you have used up all the filling.

Lightly spray the egg rolls with nonstick cooking spray. Bake for 10 to 15 minutes, or until the egg rolls are golden brown. Remove them from the oven and blot them briefly with a paper towel. Serve immediately with the Sweet and Sour Sauce. Store leftover egg rolls in an airtight container in the refrigerator for 1 to 2 days.

SHIITAKE AND CABBAGE EGG ROLLS

Well-made, non-greasy vegetable egg rolls are a real treat. For a non-vegetarian version, add some cooked chicken or pork to the filling. Egg rolls are great as appetizers; just cut the wrappers in half horizontally to make miniature versions. 🐝 **MAKES 12 EGG ROLLS**

2 ounces dry rice stick noodles

2 tablespoons grapeseed oil

1 medium red onion, cut into ¼-inch pieces (1 cup)

2 teaspoons minced garlic

1 teaspoon Aleppo pepper flakes

1 tablespoon minced fresh ginger

½ medium head white cabbage, shredded (3 cups)

½ medium head red cabbage, shredded (3 cups)

8 ounces shiitake mushrooms, stemmed and cut into ¼-inch pieces

1 teaspoon kosher salt

1 tablespoon tamari

1 tablespoon ginger-infused honey

1 tablespoon Asheville Bee Charmer's Mint-Infused Honey

2 tablespoons roughly chopped fresh mint

2 tablespoons roughly chopped fresh Thai basil

1 tablespoon roughly chopped fresh cilantro

1 (16-ounce) package egg roll wrappers

Sweet and Sour Sauce (page 179), for serving

Break the rice noodles in half and place them in a medium bowl. Pour in enough boiling water to cover them. Let the noodles sit for 10 minutes, then drain them and set aside.

In a large sauté pan over medium-high heat, heat the oil until it's hot but not yet smoking. Add the onion and garlic and cook, stirring occasionally, until the onion softens, about 5 minutes. Add the Aleppo pepper and ginger and cook for 1 minute. Add the white and red cabbages, mushrooms, and salt and cook until the cabbage softens, about 10 minutes.

Add the tamari, ginger honey, and Mint-Infused Honey and mix well. Remove the pan from the heat. Add the mint, Thai basil, cilantro, and noodles and mix well.

Preheat the oven to 425°F. Line a baking sheet with parchment paper and grease it with non-stick cooking spray.

Place an egg roll wrapper on a clean, dry surface. Wipe some water along the edges of the wrapper. Spoon about ¼ cup of the filling along one side of the wrapper, leaving an approximately 1-inch border on each side. Fold the bottom of the wrapper over the filling and then fold in the sides. Roll up the egg roll; it will look like a little burrito. Place the egg roll seam-side down on the prepared baking sheet. Repeat this process until you have used up all the filling.

Lightly spray the egg rolls with nonstick cooking spray. Bake for 10 to 15 minutes, or until the egg rolls are golden brown. Remove them from the oven and blot them briefly with a paper towel. Serve immediately with the Sweet and Sour Sauce. Store leftover egg rolls in an airtight container in the refrigerator for 1 to 2 days.

CABBAGE, GORGONZOLA, AND CANDIED WALNUT EMPANADAS

I was a vegetarian for many years, and unless I ordered a cheese empanada, I typically couldn't get a non-meat option at a restaurant. The filling for these empanadas is inspired by one of my favorite French vegetable recipes, braised red cabbage. The dandelion honey, candied walnuts, and Gorgonzola add rich flavor and just a touch of sweetness. **MAKES 25 TO 28 EMPANADAS**

DOUGH

2¼ cups all-purpose flour

1 tablespoon dried thyme

1 tablespoon dried oregano

½ teaspoon kosher salt

1 stick (½ cup) cold unsalted butter, cut into ¼-inch pieces

1 large egg

⅓ cup cold water

1 tablespoon white wine vinegar

FILLING

½ small head red cabbage, cored, quartered, and sliced ⅛ inch thick

½ large yellow onion, cut into ¼-inch cubes (about 1 cup)

1 jalapeño, seeded, deveined, and minced

½ cup water

1 tablespoon Dijon mustard

⅛ teaspoon ground cinnamon

⅛ teaspoon ground allspice

1 teaspoon kosher salt

¼ cup dandelion honey

¼ cup firmly packed light brown sugar

¾ cup Candied Walnuts (page 55), chopped

½ cup crumbled Gorgonzola cheese

EGG WASH

1 large egg

1 tablespoon warm water (about 100°F)

To make the dough, combine the flour, thyme, oregano, salt, butter, and egg in a food processor. Pulse until the mixture looks like wet sand. With the machine running, gradually add the cold water and vinegar and process until the mixture comes together. Wrap the dough in plastic wrap and refrigerate for at least 30 minutes.

In the meantime, start the filling. Place the cabbage, onion, jalapeño, water, mustard, cinnamon, allspice, salt, honey, and brown sugar in a medium saucepan set over medium-high heat. Bring the mixture to a boil. Cover the pan, reduce the heat to low, and simmer for 1 hour, or until the mixture is very soft and no longer bitter. Remove the pan from the heat, drain out the liquid, and let the mixture cool.

In a mixing bowl, combine the cooled cabbage, Candied Walnuts, and Gorgonzola.

Preheat the oven to 400°F. Line two baking sheets with parchment paper and set them aside.

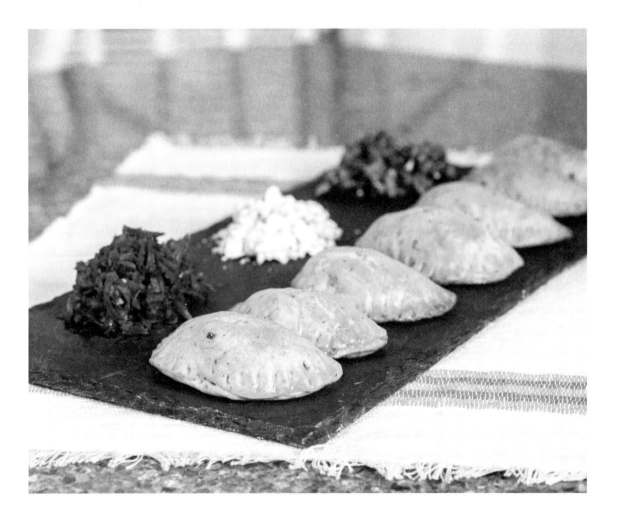

To make the egg wash, whisk together the egg and water in a small bowl.

Roll out the chilled dough to a ¼-inch thickness. Cut the dough into circles using a 2½- to 3-inch round pastry cutter. Fill each circle with approximately 1 teaspoon of the filling. Brush the edges of the circle with the egg wash. Fold over the circle to form a half moon. Seal the edges of the empanadas with a fork. Make a little slit in the top to allow steam to escape.

Place the empanadas on the prepared baking sheets, making sure they don't touch, and brush them with the egg wash. Bake for 12 to 13 minutes. Flip the empanadas, brush with the egg wash, and bake for another 12 to 13 minutes, or until they are golden brown.

Remove the empanadas from the oven and serve immediately. Store leftover empanadas in an airtight container in the refrigerator for up to 4 days or in the freezer for up to 3 months.

SPICED BEEF EMPANADAS

The twist with these empanadas is the gluten-free dough, which is made with flavorful almond flour. The combination of the almond dough and the spicy meat filling gives you a tasty appetizer or starter. The filling for these empanadas can also be used in lettuce cups or for tacos. If you manage to have any leftovers, you can refrigerate or freeze them and have them for a snack. ✿ **MAKES 25 TO 28 EMPANADAS**

DOUGH

1¾ cups almond flour

¾ cup tapioca starch

1½ teaspoons kosher salt

2 large eggs

3 tablespoons grapeseed oil

FILLING

1 tablespoon grapeseed oil

¼ medium white onion, cut into ¼-inch cubes (¼ cup)

¼ medium red bell pepper, cut into ¼-inch cubes (¼ cup)

¼ medium green bell pepper, cut into ¼-inch cubes (¼ cup)

4 ounces ground beef chuck

1 teaspoon minced garlic

1½ teaspoons Asheville Bee Charmer's Firecracker Hot Honey

¼ teaspoon red pepper flakes

¼ teaspoon paprika

¼ teaspoon ground coriander

½ teaspoon ground cumin

¼ teaspoon ancho chili powder

1 tablespoon tomato paste

½ teaspoon kosher salt

¼ teaspoon freshly ground black pepper

EGG WASH

1 large egg

1 tablespoon warm water (about 100°F)

To make the dough, combine the almond flour, tapioca starch, salt, eggs, and oil in a medium bowl and mix with a wooden spoon or spatula until well combined. If the mixture is too wet, add more almond flour, 1 teaspoon at a time. If it's too dry, add more grapeseed oil, 1 teaspoon at a time. Wrap the dough in plastic wrap and refrigerate for 10 minutes.

In the meantime, start the filling. In a large sauté pan over medium heat, heat the grapeseed oil until it's hot but not yet smoking. Add the onion and red and green bell peppers and sauté for 5 minutes, or until the onion is translucent.

Add the ground beef and garlic, breaking the meat into small pieces with a wooden spoon. Stir continuously for 5 minutes. Add the honey, pepper flakes, paprika, coriander, cumin, chili powder, tomato paste, salt, and black pepper. Mix well and cook for another 5 minutes. Remove the pan from the heat and let the filling cool completely before assembling the empanadas.

Preheat the oven to 400°F. Line two baking sheets with parchment paper and set them aside.

To make the egg wash, whisk together the egg and water in a small bowl.

Roll out the chilled dough to a ¼-inch thickness. Cut the dough into circles using a 2½- to 3-inch round pastry cutter. Fill each circle with approximately 1 teaspoon of the filling. Brush the edges of each dough circle with the egg wash. Fold over the circle to form a half moon. Seal the edges of the empanadas with a fork. Make a little slit in the top to allow steam to escape.

Place the empanadas on the prepared baking sheets, making sure they don't touch, and brush them with the egg wash. Bake for 10 to 12 minutes. Flip the empanadas, brush with the egg wash, and bake for another 10 to 12 minutes, or until they are golden brown.

Remove the empanadas from the oven and serve immediately. Store leftover empanadas in an airtight container in the refrigerator for up to 4 days or in the freezer for up to 3 months.

ASIAN DUCK CIGARS

Duck is one of my favorite proteins to cook and eat. It is prevalent in French cooking as well as in Asian cooking. This is my take on French-Asian fusion cooking. These cigars work well as a starter, but on those days when you just want something light for dinner, you can also serve them as a main course with a big salad. 🐝 **MAKES 4 CIGARS**

DUCK

2 duck legs (about 1½ pounds)

1 pound duck fat, or enough to cover the duck legs, melted

2 tablespoons grapeseed oil

1 shallot, minced

3 cloves garlic, minced

1 jalapeño, minced

12 ounces button mushrooms, sliced

2 teaspoons Asheville Bee Charmer's Ghost Pepper Honey

2 tablespoons chopped fresh flat-leaf parsley

3 teaspoons plain breadcrumbs

12 (14 × 18-inch) sheets of phyllo dough

⅓ cup unsalted butter, melted

DIPPING SAUCE

⅓ cup ketchup

⅓ cup freshly squeezed orange juice

2 teaspoons hoisin sauce

½ teaspoon oyster sauce

2 teaspoons sambal oelek

1 teaspoon Asheville Bee Charmer's Ghost Pepper Honey

Preheat the oven to 350°F. Line a baking sheet with parchment paper and set it aside.

To cook the duck, place the duck legs skin-side down in a small roasting pan. Cover with the duck fat. Transfer the pan to the oven and bake for 1½ to 2 hours, or until the duck is tender. Remove the pan from the oven and set it aside, leaving the oven on.

In a medium sauté pan set over medium-high heat, heat the grapeseed oil until it's hot but not yet smoking. Add the shallot and garlic and cook, stirring gently, for 2 to 3 minutes. Add the jalapeño and cook for 4 to 5 minutes, or until the jalapeño is softened.

Add the mushrooms and cook for about 10 minutes, or until the mushrooms have released all their water and browned nicely. Add the honey and stir well. Remove the pan from the heat, stir in the parsley, and set aside to cool.

Remove the duck legs from their cooking fat. Reserve ⅓ cup of the cooking fat and set it aside. Remove the skin from the duck legs and shred the meat.

Add the shredded duck to the cooled mushroom mixture in the sauté pan. Add the bread-crumbs and the reserved duck fat and mix well.

Lay out one sheet of phyllo dough and brush it with melted butter. Lay another sheet of phyllo on top and brush with butter. Place a third piece of phyllo on top and brush with butter. Make sure to brush the top layer with melted butter.

Place one-fourth of the duck mixture horizontally at the bottom of the phyllo stack, leaving an approximately 1-inch border on each side. Fold in the sides of the phyllo and carefully roll up the cigar. Place it on the prepared baking sheet. Repeat this process with the rest of the phyllo and duck mixture. You should end up with four cigars.

Bake for 5 to 10 minutes, or until the cigars are golden brown. Remove the cigars from the oven and let them cool.

Meanwhile, make the dipping sauce. In a small bowl, whisk together the ketchup, orange juice, hoisin sauce, oyster sauce, sambal oelek, and honey.

Cut the cigars in half on the diagonal and serve with the dipping sauce. Store leftover cigars in an airtight container in the refrigerator for 1 to 2 days. Store extra filling separately in an airtight container in the refrigerator for up to 4 days.

NOTE *You can usually get duck fat from the butcher. If you can't find any, you can use grapeseed oil instead.*

BEE Warm and BEE Green

CHAPTER 3

Soups and Salads

CURRIED CHICKEN SALAD

When I cook chicken, I always make extra so that I have a base for other dishes. It saves time and money—who doesn't love that? When I lived in London, I got hooked on curried chicken salad. The secret is having the flavors of mango chutney mixed with a spicy, delicate curry. The result is a delicious salad that's great with a bowl of mixed greens, on a sandwich, or as a filling for phyllo cups. Even if you think you don't like curry, give this a try. I bet you'll change your mind. 🐝 **MAKES 4 SERVINGS**

1–2 pieces of cooked chicken (boneless, skinless breast or thigh), chopped into ½-inch cubes (2 cups)

¼ large red onion, chopped into ¼-inch cubes (½ cup)

1 mango, peeled and chopped into ¼-inch cubes (1 cup)

½ cup raisins

½ cup salted, roasted cashews, roughly chopped

½ cup mayonnaise

3 tablespoons freshly squeezed lime juice

2 teaspoons basswood honey

2 tablespoons Madras curry powder

1 teaspoon ground ginger

1 teaspoon Aleppo pepper flakes

½ teaspoon kosher salt

¼ teaspoon freshly ground black pepper

In a medium bowl, combine the chicken, onion, mango, raisins, and cashews; set aside.

In a small bowl, whisk together the mayonnaise, lime juice, honey, curry powder, ginger, Aleppo pepper, salt, and black pepper.

Pour the curry mixture over the chicken mixture and stir gently to combine. Refrigerate for at least 30 minutes before serving. Store leftover salad in an airtight container in the refrigerator for 3 to 4 days.

KALE, CLEMENTINE, AND HAZELNUT SALAD

This is one of my favorite salads to make. It's easy and you can store it in the refrigerator. Typically, a dressed salad would wilt, but there's something interesting about this one: the longer it sits, the tastier it gets. The massaged kale is a great base for a wide range of fruits and nuts—be creative and make this salad with some of your favorites. I personally love using dried cranberries, pomegranate seeds, and toasted pecans. *MAKES 4 SERVINGS*

SALAD
1 pound curly kale, stemmed, washed, and dried thoroughly

1 tablespoon olive oil

1 tablespoon freshly squeezed lemon juice

1 teaspoon kosher salt

4 clementines, peeled and segmented

1 cup roasted hazelnuts, roughly chopped

DRESSING
3 tablespoons olive oil

2 tablespoons freshly squeezed lemon juice

2 tablespoons orange blossom honey

To make the salad, tear the kale into small pieces and place them in a large bowl. Add the olive oil, lemon juice, and salt. Gently massage the kale for 2 to 3 minutes, or until the kale has deflated by roughly half. Add the clementines and hazelnuts and toss well.

To make the dressing, whisk together the olive oil, lemon juice, and honey in a small bowl. Add the dressing to the salad and toss to coat completely. Serve the salad immediately or store it in an airtight container in the refrigerator for 4 to 5 days.

NOTE *If you don't have curly kale on hand, you can use any other kind of kale you like, including black kale, lacinato kale, Siberian kale, red Russian kale, or redbor kale.*

Pictured on p. 98

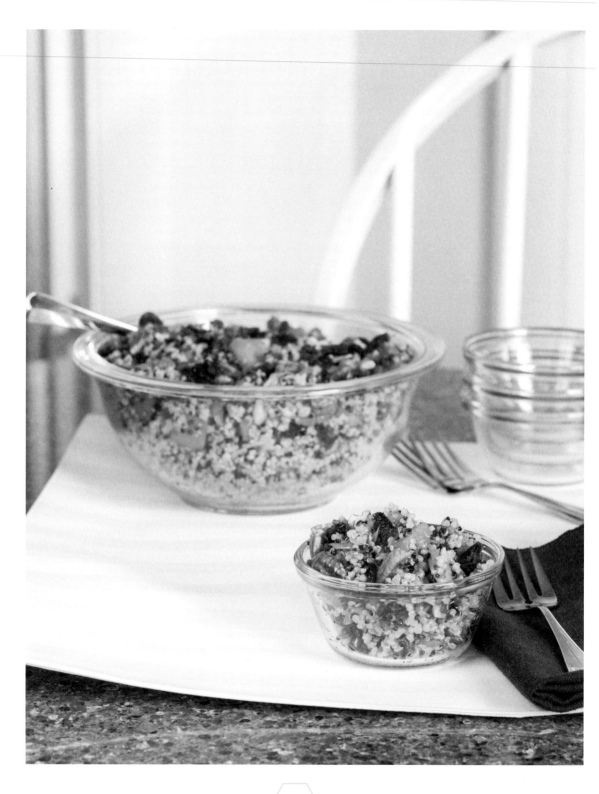

ROASTED SQUASH, QUINOA, CRANBERRY, AND PECAN SALAD

In Chicago, we have a robust winter squash season, which is great since squash is so good for you. One of my favorite ways to make squash is to roast it. All the sweetness of the fruit comes out, and if you add a little bit of honey, it adds a depth to the flavor that's hard to beat. I typically make this salad with quinoa, cranberries, and pecans. However, you can substitute your favorite grain, dried fruit, or nut. The squash is mild enough that it pairs well with a variety of other ingredients. ❧ **MAKES 6 SERVINGS**

2 tablespoons olive oil

1 tablespoon Corsican blossom honey

1 teaspoon kosher salt, divided

½ teaspoon freshly ground black pepper, divided

½ medium butternut squash, chopped into ½-inch cubes (2 cups)

2 cups water

1 cup uncooked red or white quinoa or a mix, rinsed well

1 cup unsalted, roasted pecans, roughly chopped

1 cup unsweetened dried cranberries

¼ cup Honey Mustard Vinaigrette (page 175)

3 green onions, sliced on the bias

Preheat the oven to 450°F. Line a baking sheet with parchment paper and set it aside.

In a small bowl, whisk together the olive oil, honey, ½ teaspoon of the salt, and ¼ teaspoon of the black pepper. Add the butternut squash and toss to coat completely.

Transfer the squash to the prepared baking sheet and roast for 15 minutes. Remove from the oven and stir the squash, then roast it for an additional 10 minutes, until it is golden brown and fork tender. Remove the squash from the oven and set it aside.

In a medium saucepan set over high heat, bring the water to a boil. Whisk in the quinoa, the remaining ½ teaspoon of salt, and the remaining ¼ teaspoon of black pepper. Bring the mixture back to a boil. Cover the pan, reduce the heat to low, and cook for 15 minutes. Remove the pan from the heat, still covered, and let the quinoa steam for an additional 15 minutes.

Transfer the quinoa to a large bowl. Add the roasted squash, pecans, and cranberries. Stir gently to mix. Add the Honey Mustard Vinaigrette and stir gently until everything is fully coated. Add the green onions and stir gently to combine.

Cover and refrigerate the salad until you're ready to eat. Bring it back to room temperature before serving. Store leftover salad in an airtight container in the refrigerator for 4 to 5 days.

NOTE *You can substitute kabocha squash, carnival squash, sugar or pie pumpkin, red kuri squash, buttercup squash, delicata squash, or acorn squash for the butternut squash. Or use a combination of your favorite kinds.*

APPLE PARSNIP SOUP

Parsnips, like many other root vegetables, are surprisingly sweet when you roast them. I remember the day I roasted about 5 pounds of parsnips for two people. With all those leftovers, I made this sweet and savory soup. When people try it, they are always surprised that it contains no cream. It's thick, hearty, and perfect for a cold winter night. If you want to cut a bit of the sweetness, you can substitute Granny Smith apples for the Braeburns. ❧ **MAKES 10 TO 12 SERVINGS**

¼ cup olive oil

2 tablespoons sage honey

5–6 parsnips, peeled and chopped into 1-inch cubes (5 cups)

2 tablespoons grapeseed oil

½ large yellow onion, chopped into ¼-inch cubes (1 cup)

2 cloves garlic, minced

1 tablespoon minced fresh ginger

2–3 Braeburn apples, peeled, cored, and chopped into ¼-inch cubes (3 cups)

½ teaspoon ground nutmeg

½ teaspoon kosher salt

¼ teaspoon freshly ground black pepper

1 cup unsweetened applesauce

4 cups unsalted or low-sodium vegetable stock

2 cups water

¾ cup unsalted, roasted pumpkin seeds, for garnish

Preheat the oven to 450°F. Line a baking sheet with parchment paper and set it aside.

In a measuring cup, whisk together the olive oil and sage honey. Place the parsnips in a medium bowl. Add the oil-honey mixture and toss until the parsnips are well coated. Transfer the mixture to the prepared baking sheet and roast for 15 minutes. Remove the parsnips from the oven, stir, and roast for an additional 10 minutes, or until they are lightly browned. Remove the parsnips from the oven and set them aside.

In a 6- to 8-quart stockpot set over medium-high heat, warm the grapeseed oil until it's hot but not yet smoking. Add the onion and sauté until it is soft and translucent, about 5 minutes. Add the garlic and ginger and cook for 1 minute. Add the apples, nutmeg, salt, and pepper and cook for 2 minutes. Add the parsnips, applesauce, vegetable stock, and water. Bring the liquid to a boil, reduce the heat to medium low, and simmer for 30 minutes, or until the apples and parsnips are very soft.

Remove the pot from the heat. Purée the soup either in a blender in batches, or directly in the pot with an immersion blender. Although the soup is meant to be slightly thick, you can thin it with water, if necessary. If you thin it out with water, make sure to taste it again to see if it's seasoned properly.

Ladle the soup into bowls. Top each bowl with 1 tablespoon of the roasted pumpkin seeds and serve hot. Store leftover soup in an airtight container in the refrigerator for 4 to 5 days or in the freezer for up to 6 months.

HEALTHY GARBAGE SALAD

This is my version of a garbage salad, made with ingredients I pretty much always have on hand from late summer until early spring. But it's a salad that works well with a number of ingredients. You can use a variety of hearty greens, squash, dried fruit, or beans. It is protein packed, healthy, and easy to assemble. It's great for lunch or with a roasted or grilled protein. ❧ **MAKES 8 TO 10 SERVINGS**

SALAD

¼ cup olive oil, divided

2 tablespoons carrot honey

1½ teaspoons kosher salt, divided

½ medium butternut squash, peeled and chopped into ¼-inch cubes (2 cups)

2 cups water

1 cup uncooked white or red quinoa, rinsed well

1 bunch Tuscan kale, stemmed and cut into ¼-inch slices

2 tablespoons freshly squeezed lemon juice

¼ large red onion, chopped into ¼-inch cubes (½ cup)

1–2 Gala apples, cored and chopped into ¼-inch cubes (1½ cups)

1 (15-ounce) can garbanzo beans, drained and rinsed

½ cup currants

DRESSING

2 tablespoons olive oil

2 tablespoons freshly squeezed lemon juice

1 tablespoon carrot honey

½ teaspoon kosher salt

½ teaspoon freshly ground black pepper

Preheat the oven to 450°F. Line a baking sheet with parchment paper and set it aside. To start the salad, whisk together 2 tablespoons of the oil, the honey, and ½ teaspoon of the salt in a medium bowl. Add the squash and toss to coat well. Transfer the squash to the prepared baking sheet and roast for 10 minutes. Carefully stir the squash and continue roasting for an additional 10 minutes, or until the squash is golden brown and fork tender. Remove the squash from the oven and let it cool.

In a small saucepan set over medium-high heat, bring the water to a boil. Stir in the quinoa and ½ teaspoon of the salt and bring the water back to a boil. Cover, reduce the heat to low, and simmer for 15 minutes. Remove the pan from the heat, still covered, and let the quinoa steam for 15 minutes. Spread the quinoa on a plate or baking sheet and let it cool.

Place the kale in a medium bowl. Add the remaining 2 tablespoons of oil, the lemon juice, and the remaining ½ teaspoon of salt. Massage the kale gently for 2 to 3 minutes, or until the kale has deflated by roughly half. Add the quinoa, roasted squash, and the remaining salad ingredients.

To make the dressing, whisk together all the ingredients in a small bowl. Add the dressing to the salad and stir gently with a large spoon, making sure to mix until the dressing coats all the ingredients equally. Serve the salad immediately or store it in an airtight container in the refrigerator for up to 5 days. Bring the salad back to room temperature before serving.

THAI LEMONGRASS TOFU SALAD

I learned to make this dish when I was in culinary school, and it brought back many great taste memories from my extensive travels in Thailand. The trick to using lemongrass is to make sure that you remove the really hard parts, peel and discard a couple of layers, and then mince it really finely. Typically, Thai food uses palm sugar, but I have substituted basswood honey in this version. ❧ **MAKES 4 SERVINGS**

2 stalks lemongrass, trimmed, outside layers removed, and minced

2 tablespoons tamari

1 serrano chile, seeded, deveined, and finely chopped

1 teaspoon ground turmeric

1 tablespoon basswood honey

1 teaspoon kosher salt, divided

½ cup grapeseed oil, divided

15 ounces extra-firm tofu, cut into ½-inch cubes

1 large red onion, sliced ⅛ inch thick (about 2 cups)

¼ cup minced shallots

1 clove garlic, minced

½ cup unsalted, roasted peanuts, chopped, divided

¾ cup fresh basil leaves (Thai basil if possible), cut into chiffonade, divided

3 shallots, sliced ⅛ inch thick

¼ cup all-purpose flour

6 cups baby arugula

½ cup Lemongrass Vinaigrette (page 175)

In a medium bowl, mix together the lemongrass, tamari, serrano chile, turmeric, honey, ½ teaspoon of the salt, and 1 tablespoon of the grapeseed oil. Add the tofu and mix gently, making sure that the tofu is completely and evenly coated. Cover and set aside for 1 hour.

In a large sauté pan, heat 1 tablespoon of the grapeseed oil over medium-high heat until it's hot but not yet smoking. Add the onion, minced shallots, garlic, and the remaining ½ teaspoon of salt. Cook, stirring occasionally, until the onions are translucent and starting to brown, about 10 minutes. Remove the pan from the heat and transfer the vegetables to a bowl.

In the same pan, heat 2 tablespoons of the grapeseed oil over medium-high heat until it's hot but not smoking. Add the tofu mixture and sear until the tofu is lightly browned on all sides, about 7 to 10 minutes. Add the onion mixture, ¼ cup of the peanuts, and ¼ cup of the basil. Remove the pan from the heat.

In a medium sauté pan, heat the remaining ¼ cup grapeseed oil over medium-high heat until it's hot but not yet smoking. In a small bowl, toss the shallot slices in the flour, shaking off any excess. Add the shallots to the pan and fry them in batches until lightly browned, about 2 to 3 minutes. Drain the fried shallots on paper towels.

To assemble the salad, place 1½ cups of the arugula on the center of each of four plates. Drizzle each mound of arugula with 2 tablespoons of the Lemongrass Vinaigrette. Divide the tofu among the plates, placing it on top of the arugula. Top each salad with some fried shallots. Garnish with the remaining ¼ cup of chopped peanuts and the remaining ½ cup of basil. Serve immediately.

THAI COCONUT SHRIMP SOUP

I am a year-round soup person. Hot soup in the summer can actually cool you off; it raises your internal body temperature closer to the outside temperature, which makes you feel cooler. Eating spicy food can accomplish the same thing. This soup is light, so you can eat a big bowl of it for a main course or a smaller bowl with something else for a healthy yet filling lunch or dinner. To balance the soup for your palate, play with the levels of honey, lime juice, fish sauce, and salt. Just make sure you add the salt last, as the fish sauce is salty! ❧ **MAKES 8 SERVINGS**

8 cups unsalted or low-sodium chicken stock

2 (13.5-ounce) cans coconut milk

2 stalks lemongrass, trimmed and sliced into ⅛-inch rounds

2-inch piece fresh ginger, peeled and cut into 8 (¼-inch-thick) slices

2 jalapeños, minced

1 cup roughly chopped fresh cilantro leaves and stems

Freshly grated zest of 2 limes

1 pound (26–30 count) shrimp, peeled, deveined, and tails removed

2 (15-ounce) cans straw mushrooms, drained

1 tablespoon Asheville Bee Charmer's Ghost Pepper Honey

1 tablespoon carrot honey

2 tablespoons fish sauce

¼ cup freshly squeezed lime juice

2 teaspoons kosher salt

Combine the stock and coconut milk in a 6-quart stockpot and bring the mixture to a simmer over medium-high heat. Add the lemongrass, ginger, jalapeños, cilantro, and lime zest. Reduce the heat to medium and simmer for 15 minutes.

Add the shrimp and straw mushrooms and simmer for about 2 minutes, until the shrimp just turn opaque. Add the Ghost Pepper Honey, carrot honey, fish sauce, lime juice, and salt. Stir gently until the honey disappears. Serve immediately. Store leftover soup in an airtight container in the refrigerator for 1 to 2 days.

SESAME BEEF AND ASPARAGUS SALAD

Sesame and beef make a killer flavor combination. Most recipes for sesame beef just call for the use of sesame seeds to impart flavor. I have found that using tahini adds another flavor level that can't be beat. This is a great summer dish, but you can make it all year round. This also pairs well with broccoli, green beans, or even sautéed hearty greens. ❧ **MAKES 3 TO 4 SERVINGS**

1 tablespoon yellow miso paste

1 tablespoon tahini

¼ cup tamari

¼ cup sake

1 tablespoon freshly squeezed lemon juice

1 tablespoon sesame oil

1 tablespoon ginger-infused honey

2 green onions, minced

2 tablespoons minced garlic

2 tablespoons minced fresh ginger

1 pound flank steak

¼ cup + 1 tablespoon grapeseed oil, divided

1 pound asparagus, trimmed and sliced ½ inch thick on the bias

½ teaspoon kosher salt

2 shallots, sliced ⅛ inch thick

¼ cup all-purpose flour

6 cups baby arugula

24 grape tomatoes, halved lengthwise

¾–1 cup Miso Vinaigrette (page 175)

2 green onions, sliced on the bias

To make the marinade, whisk together the miso, tahini, tamari, sake, lemon juice, sesame oil, honey, minced green onions, garlic, and ginger in a small bowl. Place the steak in a gallon-sized zip-top bag. Add the marinade and coat well. Seal the bag and let the beef marinate at room temperature for 1 hour.

Heat a grill to medium high. Wipe off the excess marinade from the steak and discard the marinade. Grill the steak for 7 to 8 minutes on each side, or until it is cooked to your liking. Remove the steak from the grill and let it rest on a plate tented with foil for at least 10 minutes.

In a medium sauté pan, heat 1 tablespoon of the grapeseed oil over medium-high heat until it's hot but not yet smoking. Add the asparagus and salt and sauté for 2 to 3 minutes, until the asparagus is cooked through but still crisp. Transfer the asparagus to a plate and set it aside.

In the same pan, heat the remaining ¼ cup of grapeseed oil over medium-high heat until it's hot but not yet smoking.

In a small bowl, toss the shallot slices in the flour, shaking off any excess. Add the shallots to the pan and fry them in small batches until lightly browned, about 2 to 3 minutes. Drain the fried shallots on paper towels.

Cut the rested flank steak against the grain into ½-inch-thick slices.

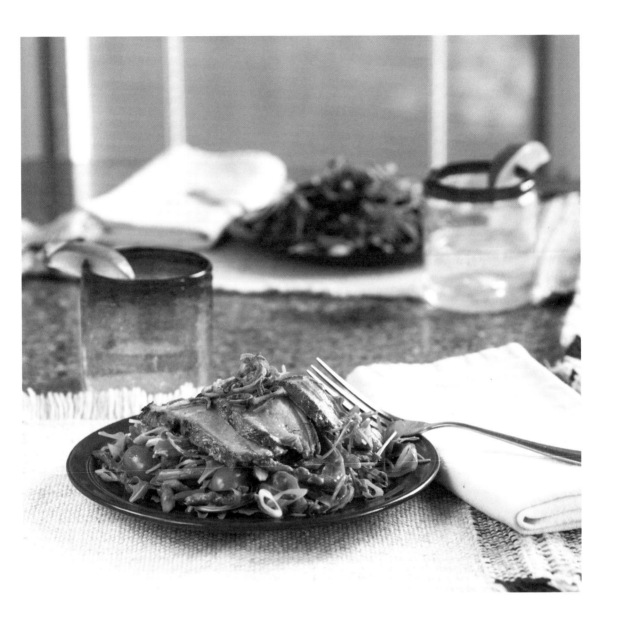

To assemble the salad, place 1½ cups of the arugula on the center of each of four plates. Put 12 tomato halves around each plate. Drizzle each mound of arugula with 2 tablespoons of the Miso Vinaigrette. Divide the asparagus among the plates, placing it on top of the arugula. Place three or four slices of steak on top of the asparagus on each plate. Brush each serving of steak with 1 to 2 tablespoons of the vinaigrette. Top each plate with some fried shallots and green onion slices. Serve immediately. Store any leftover beef in an airtight container in the refrigerator for up to 4 days or in the freezer for up to 3 months.

PUMPKIN LEEK SOUP

There are many recipes for puréed vegetable soups that use milk or cream for thickness and creamy flavor. Although those soups may taste delicious, I have always been a fan of vegetable soups that rely on their own delightful flavors to be thick, creamy, and delectable. The thickener in this soup is potato. Using vegetable stock rather than water as a cooking liquid adds yet another layer of mouthwatering flavor. **MAKES 4 TO 6 SERVINGS**

2 tablespoons grapeseed oil

3 large leeks (white and light green parts only), halved and sliced ¼ inch thick (3 cups)

½ pound russet potatoes, peeled and cut into ¼-inch cubes (about 1 cup)

1 (15-ounce) can pumpkin purée

2 teaspoons kosher salt

½ teaspoon freshly ground black pepper

2 tablespoons Corsican blossom honey

1 teaspoon ground ginger

½ teaspoon ground allspice

¼ teaspoon ground nutmeg

4 cups unsalted or low-sodium vegetable stock, divided

2 green onions, sliced ⅛ inch thick on the bias, for garnish

Heat the grapeseed oil in a small stockpot over medium heat until it's hot but not yet smoking. Add the leeks and sauté for 5 minutes, making sure they don't get any color. Add the potatoes and cook for another 5 minutes. Add the pumpkin purée, salt, black pepper, honey, ginger, allspice, and nutmeg. Cook, stirring well, for 2 minutes.

Add 3 cups of the vegetable stock and bring the liquid to a boil. Cover, reduce the heat to medium low, and simmer for 30 minutes, or until the potatoes are softened, stirring occasionally to prevent the potato and pumpkin from burning. Remove the pot from the heat and add the remaining 1 cup of vegetable stock.

Blend the soup in batches in a blender, 3 to 4 minutes per batch. Ladle the soup into four to six soup bowls. Garnish each bowl with some sliced green onion. Serve immediately. Store leftover soup in an airtight container in the refrigerator for up to 7 days or in the freezer for up to 6 months.

STRAWBERRY SPINACH SALAD

When strawberries pop up at farmers' markets in Chicago, you know that summer is just around the corner. During the short strawberry season, I try to use them in as many meals as possible. Spinach salads have been a favorite since I was a little girl, and this one is a family staple because it's loaded with strawberries. If you want to add a bit of crunch, throw in some romaine lettuce. **☞ MAKES 4 TO 6 SERVINGS**

¼ cup light mayonnaise

1 tablespoon white wine vinegar

2 tablespoons raspberry honey

2 tablespoons 2% milk

1 tablespoon poppy seeds

5 ounces baby spinach

8 ounces fresh strawberries, hulled and sliced ¼ inch thick

½ large red onion, sliced ⅛ inch thick (1 cup)

To make the dressing, whisk together the mayonnaise, vinegar, honey, milk, and poppy seeds in a small bowl; set aside.

In a large bowl, combine the spinach, strawberries, and onion. Add the dressing and toss until the salad is well coated. Serve immediately.

CURRIED SQUASH SOUP WITH SPICED PUMPKIN SEEDS

This is a simple, flavorful, healthy soup that can be served hot or cold as a starter or with some crusty bread and a salad as a light dinner. It is thick and creamy yet uses no dairy. The curry flavor is enhanced by the use of curry powder on the pumpkin seeds. *✻ MAKES 4 TO 6 SERVINGS*

SPICED PUMPKIN SEEDS

1 cup salted, roasted pumpkin seeds

1 tablespoon grapeseed oil

1 tablespoon Corsican blossom honey

1 tablespoon Madras curry powder

SOUP

2 tablespoons olive oil

1 large yellow onion, sliced ⅛ inch thick (about 2 cups)

2 tablespoons roughly chopped fresh ginger

2 cloves garlic, roughly chopped

1 tablespoon Madras curry powder

1 teaspoon kosher salt

½ teaspoon freshly ground black pepper

4 cups roasted squash purée (butternut, acorn, carnival, or any other hard winter squash; see Note)

2 tablespoons Corsican blossom honey

3 cups unsalted or low-sodium vegetable stock

1 cup carrot juice

Preheat the oven to 350°F. Line a baking sheet with parchment paper and set it aside. To make the spiced pumpkin seeds, toss them with the oil, honey, and curry powder in a small bowl, making sure all the seeds are coated. Transfer the seeds to the prepared baking sheet and bake for 15 minutes. Remove the baking sheet from the oven, transfer the seeds with the parchment paper to a cooling rack, and set aside.

To make the soup, heat the oil in a stockpot over medium-high heat until it's hot but not yet smoking. Add the onion, ginger, and garlic and cook for 10 minutes, until the onions are softened and just starting to brown. Stir in the curry powder and cook for 1 minute, until fragrant. Add the salt, pepper, squash, honey, vegetable stock, and carrot juice. Stir well and bring the liquid to a boil. Cover the pot, reduce the heat to medium low, and simmer for 20 minutes. Remove the pot from the heat.

Blend the soup in batches in a blender, 3 to 4 minutes per batch. Ladle the soup into four to six soup bowls. Garnish each bowl with 3 to 4 tablespoons of the spiced pumpkin seeds. Serve immediately. Store leftover soup in an airtight container in the refrigerator for up to 7 days or in the freezer for up to 6 months.

NOTE *You can buy canned squash purée, but it's so much better to make your own. Peel and chop any hard winter squash into 1-inch cubes. For every cup of cubed squash, toss it with 1 tablespoon of oil. Season with salt and pepper. Place the squash on a baking sheet lined with parchment paper. Roast it in a 450°F oven for 15 minutes. Stir and continue roasting for another 10 minutes, or until the squash is fork tender. Place the roasted squash with a little bit of water in a blender and purée until smooth.*

CITRUS SPINACH SALAD

The acidity in citrus complements the mineral notes of spinach, making this culinary duo one of my favorites. I like to use clementine, but you can substitute orange, pomelo, mandarin, tangerine, kumquat, or grapefruit, if you prefer. Eat this salad right away—once it's dressed, the spinach will wilt and become soggy very quickly. *MAKES 4 SERVINGS*

1 teaspoon minced shallot

1 clove garlic, minced

1 tablespoon freshly squeezed lemon juice

1 tablespoon orange blossom honey

1 teaspoon freshly grated orange zest

½ teaspoon kosher salt

¼ teaspoon freshly ground black pepper

2 tablespoons olive oil

¼ medium red onion, thinly sliced

3 clementines, peeled and segmented

¼ cup unsalted, roasted almonds, roughly chopped

5 ounces baby spinach

To make the dressing, whisk together the shallot, garlic, lemon juice, honey, orange zest, salt, and pepper in a small bowl. Slowly whisk in the olive oil until fully emulsified. Set the dressing aside.

In a large bowl, combine the spinach, red onion, clementines, and almonds. Add the dressing and toss until the salad is well coated. Serve immediately.

PIÑAPRESE

A few years ago, I worked on making a variation of a traditional caprese salad. After some trial and error, this tropical-flavored recipe was the result. Instead of tomato, I used pineapple and red bell pepper, roasted to enhance its natural sweetness. The pesto adds the basil element, plus a hint of spiciness that balances the sweetness. Add the creaminess of the mozzarella, and you have a great salad that works any time of the year. 🐝 **MAKES 4 SERVINGS**

PESTO

1 cup pine nuts

3 cloves garlic

2 serrano chiles, seeded and deveined

4 cups tightly packed fresh basil leaves

½ teaspoon kosher salt

¼ teaspoon freshly ground black pepper

¾ cup olive oil, plus more for brushing

1 cup grated Parmigiano-Reggiano

CROSTINI AND PIÑAPRESE

4 slices baguette, sliced 5 inches long on the bias and ¼ inch thick

1 tablespoon grapeseed oil

1 tablespoon tupelo honey

¼ pineapple, cored and sliced into 8 (¼-inch-thick) pieces

2 red bell peppers, roasted and peeled

12 ounces fresh mozzarella

Preheat the oven to 350°F. Line two baking sheets with parchment paper and set them aside.

To make the pesto, add the pine nuts, garlic, serrano chiles, basil, salt, and pepper to the bowl of a food processor and process until chopped. With the motor running, slowly add the ¾ cup of the olive oil. Continue processing until the mixture is well combined but still has some texture. Transfer the pesto to a bowl and stir in the Parmigiano-Reggiano. Set aside.

To make the crostini, brush both sides of the baguette slices with the olive oil and place them on one of the prepared baking sheets. Bake the bread for 10 minutes, flipping the slices halfway through, until golden brown. Remove the baking sheet from the oven and set it aside. Increase the oven temperature to 400°F.

In a small bowl, whisk together the grapeseed oil and honey. Brush the pineapple slices on both sides with the mixture and transfer them to the second prepared baking sheet. Roast, flipping halfway through, for 20 minutes, or until they are lightly browned. Remove the baking sheet from the oven and set it aside.

Cut each roasted red pepper into four squares. Cut the mozzarella into 12 (1-ounce) slices.

To assemble the salad, layer equal amounts of the pepper, pineapple, and mozzarella among four plates, making sure to position a slice of cheese between each fruit and vegetable slice. Each plate should have a total of two pepper squares, two pineapple slices, and three mozzarella slices. Drizzle each plate with ¼ cup of the pesto. Add one crostini to each plate and serve. Store leftover components of the salad separately in airtight containers in the refrigerator for 3 to 4 days.

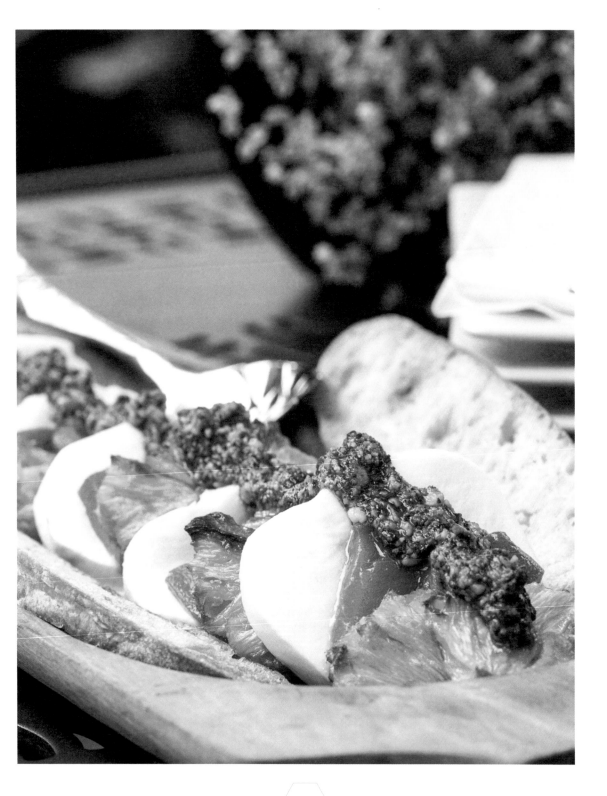

the asheville bee charmer cookbook

MOROCCAN CARROT SOUP

I seem to always have extra carrots in the house. Although I like to use them in baked goods, I also use them in soup. The Moroccan spices in this soup add a lot of depth to the natural sweetness of the carrots. Although the soup doesn't use any dairy, I use Greek yogurt as a garnish because it provides a lovely contrast to the spices. If you want to keep the soup dairy free, use unsweetened plain coconut yogurt as a substitute. **MAKES 6 TO 8 SERVINGS**

3 tablespoons olive oil

12 medium carrots, cut into ½-inch cubes (6 cups)

1 large yellow onion, cut into ½-inch cubes (about 2 cups)

4 cloves garlic, roughly chopped

1 (1-inch) piece fresh ginger, peeled and roughly chopped

1 teaspoon ground cumin

1 teaspoon ground ginger

1 teaspoon kosher salt

1 teaspoon Aleppo pepper flakes

½ teaspoon ground coriander

½ teaspoon ground allspice

¼ teaspoon ground cloves

1 tablespoon Asheville Bee Charmer's Firecracker Hot Honey

1 tablespoon ginger-infused honey

6 cups unsalted or low-sodium vegetable stock, divided

¾–1 cup plain Greek yogurt, for garnish

¼ cup minced fresh cilantro, for garnish

In a medium stockpot, heat the olive oil over medium-high heat until it's hot but not smoking. Add the carrots and onion and cook, stirring occasionally, for about 10 minutes, or until the vegetables are lightly browned.

Add the garlic, fresh ginger, cumin, ground ginger, salt, Aleppo pepper flakes, coriander, allspice, cloves, Firecracker Hot Honey, and ginger honey. Stir well and cook for 2 to 3 minutes. Add 4 cups of the vegetable stock and bring it to a boil. Cover the pot, reduce the heat to medium low, and simmer for 20 minutes, or until the carrots are fully softened. Remove the pot from the heat and stir in the remaining 2 cups of vegetable stock.

Blend the soup in batches in a blender, 3 to 4 minutes per batch. Ladle the soup into six to eight soup bowls. Garnish each bowl with some yogurt and minced cilantro. Serve immediately. Store leftover soup in an airtight container in the refrigerator for up to 7 days or in the freezer for up to 6 months.

NOTE *This soup is thick; the yogurt garnish makes it thinner. However, if you want, you can add some water, 1 to 2 tablespoons at a time, until it's the consistency that you like. Make sure to check the seasoning again before serving. This also makes a great cold soup. If you plan to serve it cold, cool it for about 1 hour at room temperature before refrigerating.*

CORN CHOWDER

Although corn is a wonderful summer vegetable, there is nothing like enjoying hearty corn chowder during the colder months of the year. If you can't get fresh vegetables, the next best thing is frozen vegetables, as they have been picked at peak ripeness and flash frozen. Just check to make sure there is nothing added to the vegetables you're buying. Although this soup uses Mexican spices, it isn't hot; it's just flavorful. If you want to add heat, use the poblano seeds and veins. The potato thickens the chowder. The recipe calls for a yogurt garnish, but if you want to keep it dairy free, use unsweetened plain coconut yogurt instead. ❧ **MAKES 6 TO 8 SERVINGS**

2 tablespoons grapeseed oil

2 stalks celery, cut into ¼-inch cubes

1 large yellow onion, cut into ¼-inch cubes (about 2 cups)

1 poblano chile, seeded, deveined, and cut into ¼-inch cubes

2 cloves garlic, minced

2 tablespoons sourwood honey

2 teaspoons kosher salt

1 teaspoon freshly ground black pepper

1 teaspoon ground cumin

½ teaspoon ground coriander

1 pound russet potatoes, peeled and cut into ¼-inch cubes

1 (16-ounce) bag frozen roasted corn, divided (about 3½ cups)

4 cups unsalted or low-sodium vegetable stock, divided

¼ cup roughly chopped fresh cilantro, for garnish

½ cup plain Greek yogurt, for garnish

In a medium stockpot, heat the grapeseed oil over medium-high heat until it's hot but not yet smoking. Add the celery, onion, poblano chile, and garlic. Sauté, stirring occasionally, for 10 minutes, until the vegetables are softened and just starting to color.

Add the honey, salt, pepper, cumin, and coriander and cook for 1 minute, until fragrant. Add the potatoes and half of the corn and cook, stirring occasionally, for 5 minutes. Add 3 cups of the vegetable stock and bring it to a boil. Cover the pot, reduce the heat to medium low, and simmer for 30 minutes, or until the potatoes are completely softened.

Remove the pot from the heat and add the remaining 1 cup of vegetable stock. Blend the soup in batches in a blender, 3 to 4 minutes per batch. Stir in the remaining corn. Ladle the soup into six to eight soup bowls. Garnish each serving with some chopped cilantro and Greek yogurt. Serve immediately. Store leftover soup in an airtight container in the refrigerator for up to 7 days or in the freezer for up to 6 months.

NOTE *If frozen roasted corn is unavailable, you can use plain frozen corn. If it's summer, use fresh corn kernels, either plain or roasted.*

ROASTED BEETS WITH HONEY CHIVE GOAT CHEESE

 GF V

Beets and goat cheese are a classic combination. The twist in this dish is the Corsican blossom honey, used for both roasting the beets and seasoning the goat cheese. Adding the yogurt to the goat cheese gives it more of a mousse-like quality. I often make this recipe when my chive blossoms first bloom. After the blossoms are gone, I incorporate the chives. ❀ **MAKES 3 SERVINGS**

2 tablespoons olive oil

2 tablespoons Corsican blossom honey, divided

3 medium red beets, trimmed and peeled

4 ounces plain fresh goat cheese, at room temperature

4 ounces plain Greek yogurt

¼ cup finely chopped chives and chive flowers

½ teaspoon kosher salt

¼ teaspoon freshly ground black pepper

Chive flowers and/or micro greens, for garnish

Preheat the oven to 400°F. Line a baking sheet with parchment paper and set it aside.

In a small bowl, whisk together the olive oil and 1 tablespoon of the honey. Rub the oil mixture all over the beets. Wrap each beet with aluminum foil and place it on the prepared baking sheet. Transfer the baking sheet to the oven and roast the beets for 1 hour, or until a knife can easily cut through the beets. Remove the beets from the oven and let them cool. Once they are cool enough to handle, cut each beet into eight chunks, or cut into ¼-inch slices; set aside.

In a small bowl, mix together the goat cheese, the yogurt, the remaining 1 tablespoon of honey, the chopped chives, the salt, and the pepper.

Divide the cheese mixture among three plates. Place the beets around the cheese. Garnish with the chive flowers and/or micro greens. Serve immediately. Store any leftover components separately in airtight containers in the refrigerator for 4 to 5 days.

NOTE *You can also make this dish into a tartine. Get some fresh crusty bread, like a baguette, and spread the cheese mixture on it. Top with the beets, micro greens, and chive flowers. The cheese mixture is also great on bagels with smoked salmon.*

HEARTY GREENS SLAW

A good slaw can be made of shredded cabbage, but when you use hearty greens, you create a *great* slaw. Use as many or as few varieties of greens as you like. Massaging the slaw with the dressing is a bit messy, but it's a critical step, as it rids some of the bitterness from the greens. This slaw holds up well in the refrigerator for a few days—unless you use a lot of spinach, which wilts easily. ✻ **MAKES 4 SERVINGS**

2 ounces Swiss chard or spinach leaves, julienned

2 ounces baby arugula

2 ounces kale or mustard green leaves, julienned

1 medium carrot, grated (½ cup)

2 green onions, sliced ⅛ inch thick on the bias

2 tablespoons rice vinegar

1 tablespoon sesame oil

½ tablespoon grapeseed oil

½ tablespoon Tasmanian leatherwood honey

½ teaspoon sambal oelek

1 teaspoon tahini

To make the slaw, combine the chard, arugula, kale, carrot, and green onions in a large bowl.

To make the dressing, whisk together the vinegar, sesame oil, grapeseed oil, honey, sambal oelek, and tahini in a small bowl until well emulsified.

Add the dressing to the slaw. Massage the slaw gently for about 2 to 3 minutes, or until it has deflated by roughly half. Cover and refrigerate until you're ready to serve.

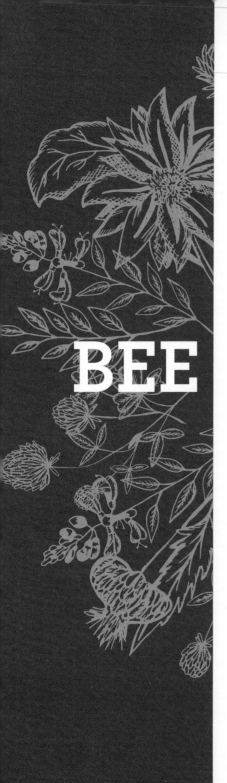

BEE Full

CHAPTER 4

Sandwiches and Mains

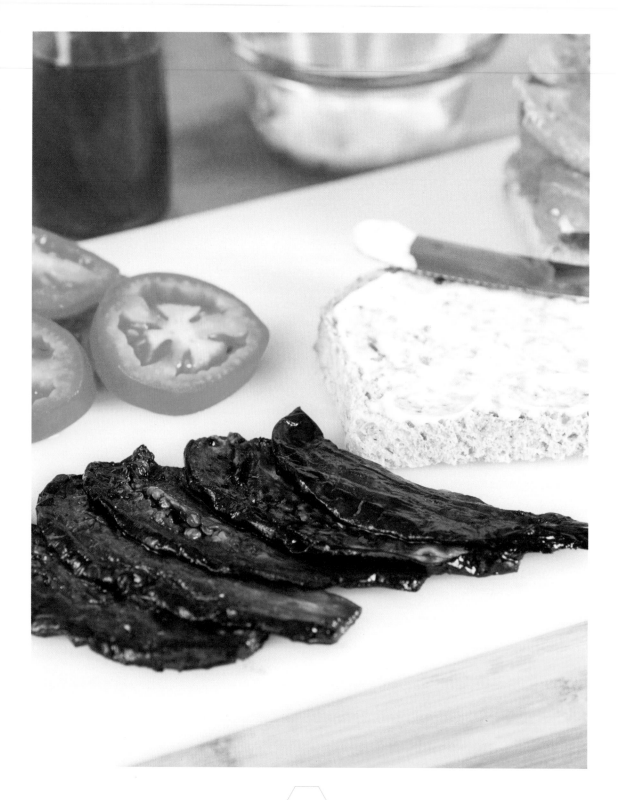

ELT

I find it satisfying to eat something that is both sweet and salty, like honey-cured bacon or choc-olate-covered pretzels. While teaching at a vegetarian cooking school called The Kids' Table, my colleagues and I developed a vegetarian version of a BLT, using savory eggplant bacon. Here, I have modified it to mimic the taste of honey-cured bacon. The addition of smoky chipotle honey on the sandwich adds a layer of flavor that will leave you wanting more. ✺ **MAKES 4 SANDWICHES**

EGGPLANT BACON

1 (1-pound) eggplant

¼ cup olive oil

3 tablespoons tamari

3 tablespoons basswood honey

MAYONNAISE

1 large egg

1 tablespoon freshly squeezed lemon juice

1 teaspoon Dijon mustard

½ teaspoon kosher salt

¼ teaspoon ground white pepper

1 cup grapeseed oil

¼ cup Asheville Bee Charmer's Smokin' Hot Honey (chipotle-infused honey)

SANDWICH ASSEMBLY

8 slices whole wheat or multigrain bread

8 leaves romaine lettuce

4 small plum tomatoes, sliced ½ inch thick

Preheat the oven to 450°F. Line a baking sheet with parchment paper and set it aside.

To make the eggplant bacon, halve the eggplant lengthwise and cut each half into ¼-inch slices. Lightly brush both sides of the eggplant slices with the olive oil. Arrange the slices in a single layer on the prepared baking sheet. Bake for 10 minutes, or until browned on top. Flip the slices and bake them on the other side for 10 minutes, or until browned. Remove the eggplant from the oven and set it aside to cool for 5 to 10 minutes on the baking sheet. Keep the oven on while you make the marinade.

To make the marinade, whisk together the tamari and basswood honey in a small bowl. Brush each side of the eggplant slices with the honey-tamari mixture and return them to the oven. Bake until crispy, about 5 minutes. Remove the eggplant from the oven and set it aside to cool. Cut each piece of eggplant lengthwise into 1-inch-thick slices.

To make the mayonnaise, place the egg, lemon juice, mustard, salt, and pepper in the bowl of a food processor. With the motor running, slowly add the oil and let process until the mixture has emulsified and thickened. Transfer ¼ cup of the mayonnaise to a small bowl (reserve the rest for another use). Whisk in the Smokin' Hot Honey.

To assemble the sandwiches, lightly toast the bread. Spread 1 tablespoon of the mayonnaise on one side of each bread slice. Place two romaine leaves on top of the mayonnaise on each of four slices. Divide the tomato slices and eggplant bacon evenly among the sandwiches. Top with the remaining bread slices (mayonnaise-side down). Serve immediately. Store leftover eggplant in an airtight container in the refrigerator for 4 to 5 days.

BRAISED GARBANZOS AND CHICKEN SAUSAGE

I've spent a lot of time in Spain, and one of my favorite country dishes is braised garbanzos with fresh pork sausage. To make it a bit healthier, I started using chicken sausage and found that the chicken, apples, and rosemary honey lend a slight sweetness to the stew that is a pleasant contrast to the garbanzo beans. You can substitute pork sausage in the stew; either mild or spicy will work. ❧ **MAKES 4 TO 5 SERVINGS**

2 tablespoons olive oil

12 ounces chicken-apple sausage, cut into ½-inch slices on the bias

1 large yellow onion, chopped into ¼-inch cubes (2 cups)

2 medium carrots, chopped into ¼-inch cubes (1 cup)

1 teaspoon dried thyme

1 teaspoon kosher salt

1 tablespoon Asheville Bee Charmer's Rosemary-Infused Honey

2 cups garbanzo beans, cooked and drained (if using canned, make sure to rinse them)

1 cup water

In a large saucepan, heat the olive oil over high heat until it's hot but not yet smoking. Add the sausage slices and cook them for 1 to 2 minutes per side, until browned. Using a slotted spoon, transfer the sausage to a small bowl; set aside.

Return the same saucepan to the stove over medium-high heat. Add the onion, carrots, thyme, and salt and cook, stirring occasionally, until the vegetables are soft, about 10 minutes. Add the honey, garbanzo beans, reserved sausage, and water. Bring the liquid to a boil, cover the pan, reduce the heat to low, and simmer for 30 minutes.

Serve with a salad and some crusty bread. Store leftover beans and sausage in an airtight container in the refrigerator for up to 4 days or in the freezer for up to 3 months.

RAGIN' ASIAN RIBS

To brine or not to brine? That is often the question amongst rib lovers. I like to use highly spiced brine for my ribs because it infuses them with tons of flavor and helps them stay moist despite the long cooking time. Additionally, I prefer to almost fully cook the ribs before I add the glaze. Don't worry—you'll have plenty of glaze left over to use as a dipping sauce for the ribs! ❧ **MAKES 4 SERVINGS**

2 gallons water

1 cup tupelo honey

1 cup kosher salt

3 tablespoons whole black peppercorns

3 tablespoons red pepper flakes

2 teaspoons dried thyme

5 cloves garlic

1 cinnamon stick

2 bay leaves

Peel of 2 oranges

2 racks pork spare ribs (6–8 pounds), each cut in half

1 cup ketchup

1 cup freshly squeezed orange juice

2 tablespoons hoisin sauce

½ tablespoon oyster sauce

2 tablespoons sambal oelek

To make the brine, mix together the water, honey, salt, peppercorns, red pepper flakes, thyme, garlic, cinnamon, bay leaves, and orange peel in a large stockpot. Add the ribs. Cover and refrigerate overnight.

Remove the ribs from the brine and pat them dry. Set them aside and let them come to room temperature. Discard the brine. Heat a grill to low.

Grill the ribs, turning frequently, for 1½ hours, or until tender. Remove the ribs from the grill and cover the grill grates with aluminum foil.

While the ribs cook, make the glaze. In a medium bowl, whisk together the ketchup, orange juice, hoisin sauce, oyster sauce, and sambal oelek; set aside.

Return the ribs to the grill and brush them with the glaze. Grill the ribs for another 30 minutes, glazing them two more times. Remove the ribs from the grill and serve with any leftover glaze. Store leftover ribs in an airtight container in the refrigerator for up to 4 days.

HONEY MUSTARD GLAZED HALIBUT

My favorite fish to eat is probably halibut. It isn't in season for very long and can be expensive, but it's worth the occasional splurge. The honey mustard glaze gives a sweet and spicy flavor to the fish. If you can't find halibut or want to use a less expensive fish, substitute grouper, cod, or any other mild, meaty fish. This recipe also works well with wild-caught salmon. **MAKES 4 SERVINGS**

¼ cup acacia honey

¼ cup Dijon mustard

2 tablespoons olive oil

1 tablespoon freshly squeezed lemon juice

4 (6-ounce) halibut fillets, boned and skinned

Kosher salt and ground white pepper, to taste

2 tablespoons grapeseed oil

Preheat the oven to 350°F.

To make the honey mustard glaze, whisk together the honey, mustard, olive oil, and lemon juice in a small bowl; set aside.

Season the fish fillets with salt and pepper. Brush the halibut all over with the glaze and set the extra glaze aside.

In a large, ovenproof sauté pan, heat the grapeseed oil over high heat until it's hot but not yet smoking. Add the halibut fillets and sear until they are golden brown, 2 to 3 minutes. Flip the fillets and place the sauté pan in the oven. Bake for 4 to 6 minutes, or until the halibut is opaque. Remove the pan from the oven and brush the fillets with the reserved honey mustard glaze. Serve immediately. Store leftover fish in an airtight container in the refrigerator for 1 to 2 days.

HONEY MUSTARD AND HERB RACK OF LAMB

This is an elegant dish that is surprisingly easy to make. A traditional French preparation is to brush a seared rack with mustard and then encrust it with an herb-breadcrumb mixture. I've found that cumin is a great spice to use with lamb, and adding it to a relatively traditional herb mixture provides a unique flavor. The addition of honey to the mustard brings sweetness to the lamb, similar to what a mint sauce might accomplish. I skip the breadcrumbs so the pure taste of the herbs can shine through. ❧ **MAKES 4 SERVINGS**

2 (1½-pound) full racks of lamb, frenched
2 tablespoons olive oil
2 teaspoons kosher salt
1 teaspoon freshly ground black pepper
1 teaspoon dried parsley
1 teaspoon dried thyme

1 teaspoon dried rosemary
½ teaspoon garlic powder
½ teaspoon ground cumin
2 tablespoons Dijon mustard
2 teaspoons Asheville Bee Charmer's
    Mint-Infused Honey

Preheat the oven to 400°F. Line a baking sheet with aluminum foil and set it aside.

Heat a large skillet over medium-high heat until it's hot but not smoking. Rub each rack of lamb with 1 tablespoon of the olive oil. Season each rack with 1 teaspoon of the salt and ½ teaspoon of the pepper.

Add the racks to the skillet, fat-side down, and sear for about 3 minutes, or until they are dark golden brown on the bottom. Flip the racks over and sear them on the other side for 3 minutes. Then, sear the ends for about 3 minutes each. Remove the racks from the heat and place them, fat-side up, on the prepared baking sheet. Let the lamb racks rest for 10 to 15 minutes.

In the meantime, mix together the parsley, thyme, rosemary, garlic powder, and cumin in a small bowl until well incorporated. Set aside.

In another small bowl, whisk together the mustard and honey. Brush the honey-mustard mixture on each rack of lamb, covering it completely. Sprinkle the herb mixture on top of the mustard.

Transfer the lamb to the oven and roast for 20 to 25 minutes, or until an instant-read thermometer registers 130°F (for medium rare) when inserted into the thickest part of the meat.

Remove the meat from the oven and let it rest for about 10 minutes on a plate tented with foil. To serve, cut the rack along the bones to make individual chops. Divide the chops evenly among four plates. Store leftover lamb in an airtight container in the refrigerator for up to 4 days.

MISO HONEY GLAZED SALMON

I learned how to make miso glazed cod in culinary school. After trying it, I was absolutely hooked on the flavor profile. Most miso glazes need to be cooked, as they contain sugar, but using honey eliminates this step. I like to use this on salmon, but it also works on cod, grouper, or any other mild, meaty fish, and it's great on chicken, too. This dish is elegant enough to serve at a dinner party, yet easy enough to make any day of the week. **MAKES 4 SERVINGS**

¼ cup sake

¼ cup mirin

¼ cup white or light yellow miso paste

¼ cup acacia honey

1½ pounds wild-caught salmon, portioned into 4 (6-ounce) fillets

Preheat the broiler with a rack 6 inches from the heat source. Line a baking sheet with aluminum foil and set it aside.

To make the marinade, in a small bowl, whisk together the sake, mirin, miso, and honey until no lumps remain. Place the salmon fillets, skin-side down, on the prepared baking sheet. Brush the salmon fillets with the marinade.

Place the salmon under the broiler for 6 to 8 minutes, or until the salmon is browned on top and still slightly dark pink in the center. If the top browns too quickly, move the baking sheet to a lower rack and continue cooking until the salmon is done to your liking. Remove the salmon from the oven and serve immediately. I prefer salmon that is medium rare, but if you like it well done, cook it for an additional 1 to 2 minutes. Make sure not to overcook it, as it dries out very quickly. Store leftover salmon in an airtight container in the refrigerator for 3 to 4 days.

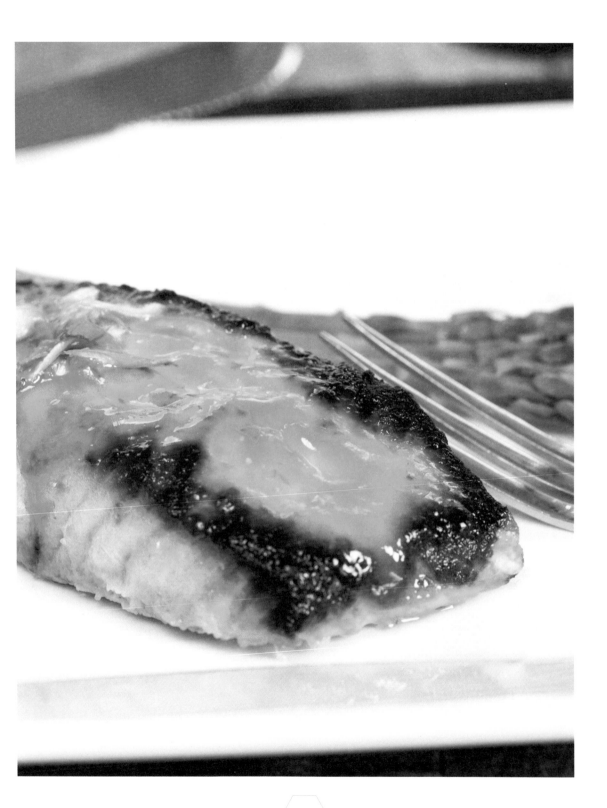

GRILLED CHEESE WITH CRANBERRY AND GHOST PEPPER

Grilled cheese, especially made with cheddar, is one of those sandwiches that remind me of my childhood. As I have gotten older, I have used more sophisticated cheeses, but my favorite remains cheddar. Last year right after Thanksgiving, I was trying to think of something to make with leftover Cranberry Orange Sauce. I decided to try it on grilled cheese, and for some additional zing, I added Ghost Pepper Honey as well. It became my favorite way to make grilled cheese. I hope it becomes one of your favorites, too. **MAKES 4 SANDWICHES**

¼ cup unsalted butter, at room temperature

8 slices whole wheat or multigrain bread

¾–1 cup Cranberry Orange Sauce (page 174)

¼ cup Asheville Bee Charmer's Ghost Pepper Honey

8 ounces sharp cheddar, grated

Butter one side of each bread slice with the butter. Lay the bread on a cutting board or piece of parchment paper, buttered-side down. Spread each of four bread slices with 3 to 4 tablespoons of the Cranberry Orange Sauce. Spread each of the remaining four slices with 1 tablespoon of the honey.

Add 2 ounces of the grated cheddar to each bread slice with cranberry sauce. Top with the other four slices of bread, buttered side up.

Heat a griddle or large saucepan over medium heat. Cook the sandwiches for 3 to 4 minutes on one side, or until golden brown. Flip and cook for another 3 to 4 minutes, or until the second side is golden brown and the cheese has melted. Serve immediately.

HONEY GLAZED ASIAN DUCK

I still remember the first time I ate Peking duck in Asia, almost 30 years ago. It is delectable to eat, but it is labor intensive to make. This version has a similar flavor profile to Peking duck but requires about one-tenth the amount of work. The marinade can burn very easily while cooking, so be careful to wipe off any excess marinade from the duck, and watch the heat on the pan. *MAKES 4 SERVINGS*

4 duck breasts (about 2 pounds), trimmed of excess fat

3 tablespoons tamari

2 tablespoons rice vinegar

2 tablespoons carrot honey

1 tablespoon grapeseed oil

1 tablespoon red pepper flakes

1 tablespoon Chinese five-spice powder

Wash and dry the duck breasts. Using a small, sharp knife, score the skin of the duck by making shallow incisions in a crosshatch pattern across the entire breast. Make sure not to cut into the flesh of the duck. Place the duck breasts in a gallon-sized zip-top bag; set aside.

To make the marinade, whisk together the tamari, vinegar, honey, grapeseed oil, red pepper flakes, and Chinese five-spice powder in a small bowl. Add the marinade to the bag with the duck breasts and coat the duck well. Seal the bag and let the duck marinate at room temperature for 1 hour.

Wipe off the excess marinade from the duck and discard the marinade. Place the duck breasts skin-side down in a large, cold sauté pan. Place a second sauté pan on top of the duck and weight it down with a metal can. Cook the duck over medium-low heat for about 10 minutes, until all the fat is rendered and the skin is brown and crispy. Remove the weight and the second pan. Drain off the extra fat and discard it or reserve it for another use.

Increase the heat to medium high and flip the duck. Cook for 6 minutes, or until an instant-read thermometer registers 135°F when inserted into the thickest part of the breast. Transfer the duck to a warm plate and let it rest for at least 5 minutes. Slice the duck at an angle against the grain and serve immediately. Store leftover duck in an airtight container in the refrigerator for up to 4 days.

NOTE *I always keep a mason jar on hand to store excess rendered duck fat in. I use it to roast or fry potatoes.*

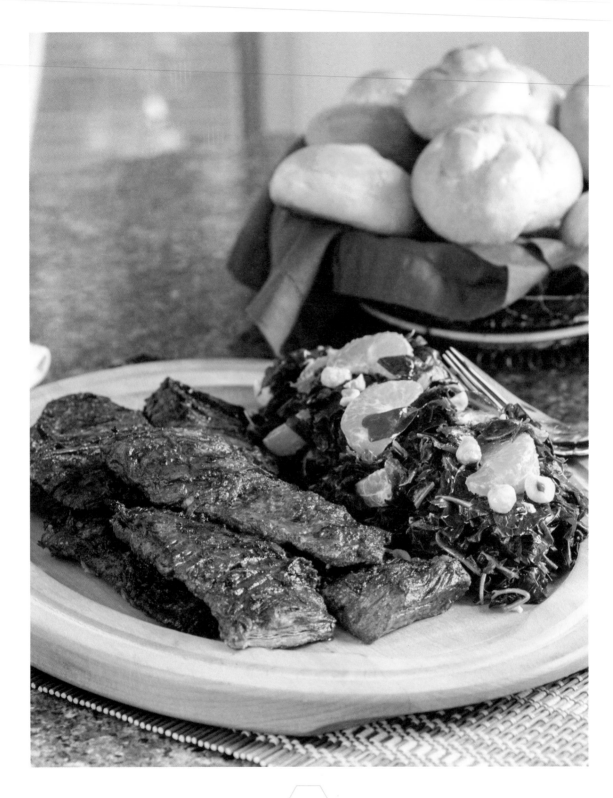

CHIPOTLE HONEY MARINATED SKIRT STEAK

I was introduced to chipotle, or smoke-dried jalapeño, as a young girl, and that hot, smoky flavor has been one of my favorites ever since. Although this marinade uses both chipotles and chipotle honey, the resulting steak isn't overly spicy; it's just really flavorful. The meat only needs to marinate for an hour, but it can marinate for up to 24 hours if you have the time. ✿ **MAKES 5 TO 6 SERVINGS**

2 tablespoons freshly squeezed lime juice

¼ large yellow onion, chopped into ¼-inch cubes (½ cup)

1½ tablespoons minced garlic

3 chipotle chiles, chopped into ¼-inch cubes

2 tablespoons Asheville Bee Charmer's Smokin' Hot Honey (chipotle-infused honey)

2 teaspoons ground cumin

2 teaspoons kosher salt

1 teaspoon ancho chili powder

1 teaspoon smoked paprika

¼ cup olive oil

2½ pounds skirt steak, cut into 2 to 3 pieces

To make the marinade, mix together the lime juice, onion, garlic, chipotle chiles, honey, cumin, salt, ancho chili powder, smoked paprika, and olive oil in a small bowl until well incorporated. Place the steak in a gallon-sized zip-top bag. Add the marinade and coat the steak well. Seal the bag and let the steak marinate at room temperature for 1 hour.

Heat a grill to medium-high heat. Wipe off the excess marinade from the steak and discard the marinade. Grill the steak for 6 to 7 minutes on each side, or until it is cooked to your liking.

Transfer the meat to a plate, tent it with foil, and let it rest for 10 minutes. Cut the steak at an angle against the grain into ¼-inch- or ½-inch-thick slices. Serve immediately. Store leftover steak in an airtight container in the refrigerator for up to 4 days or in the freezer for up to 3 months.

NOTE *If you don't have a grill, you can cook the steak under a broiler.*

Pictured at left, from top: Milk and Honey Dinner Rolls (p. 135); Kale, Clementine, and Hazelnut Salad (p. 67); Chipotle Honey Marinated Skirt Steak

MARGARITA CHICKEN THIGHS

My go-to cocktail is a margarita. It's refreshing, especially on a hot day. I wanted to bring that flavor profile, without the excessive sweetness, to a chicken dish. The tequila and triple sec tenderize the chicken, but the alcohol burns off as you cook it. All you're left with is great flavor. The Firecracker Hot Honey replaces the sugar in a margarita, but it also adds a spicy kick. I use chicken thighs whenever possible, as they are the most flavorful part of the chicken. *MAKES 4 TO 6 SERVINGS*

¼ cup silver tequila

1 tablespoon triple sec

2 tablespoons freshly squeezed lime juice

1½ tablespoons Asheville Bee Charmer's Firecracker Hot Honey

1 teaspoon kosher salt

1 clove garlic, minced

8 skin-on, boneless thighs, trimmed of excess fat

2 tablespoons grapeseed oil

To make the marinade, whisk together the tequila, triple sec, lime juice, honey, salt, and garlic in a small bowl. Place the chicken in a gallon-sized zip-top bag. Add the marinade and coat the chicken well. Seal the bag and let the chicken marinate at room temperature for 1 hour.

Preheat the oven to 350°F.

Heat the oil in a large ovenproof sauté pan over medium-high heat until it's hot but not yet smoking. Wipe off the excess marinade from the chicken and discard the marinade. Add the chicken thighs to the sauté pan, skin-side down, and sear for 3 to 4 minutes, or until golden brown. Flip the chicken and cook for another 3 to 4 minutes.

Transfer the pan to the oven and bake the chicken for 20 minutes, or until an instant-read thermometer registers 165°F when inserted into the thickest part of a thigh. Remove the pan from the oven and let the chicken rest for 5 minutes before serving. Store leftover chicken in an airtight container in the refrigerator for up to 4 days or in the freezer for up to 3 months.

SESAME CRUSTED TUNA

This dish goes from fridge to table in less than 30 minutes, even if you make a couple sides. It is elegant enough for guests and easy enough to make any day of the week. I love to pair this with Hearty Greens Slaw (page 85) or a quick stir-fry. ❧ **MAKES 4 SERVINGS**

4 (6-ounce) ahi or yellowfin tuna steaks

1 teaspoon kosher salt

¼ cup white sesame seeds

¼ cup black sesame seeds

2 tablespoons grapeseed oil

Asian Dipping Sauce (page 177), for serving

Rinse the tuna steaks, pat them dry, and season with the salt on both sides.

Mix together the white and black sesame seeds in a flat bowl or on a shallow plate. Place the tuna steaks on the dish and fully coat them in sesame seeds on all sides so that no flesh is showing. Set the coated tuna steaks aside.

In a large sauté pan, heat the oil over medium-high heat until it's hot but not yet smoking. Add the tuna steaks and sear for 1 to 2 minutes on each side, or until golden brown (for rare tuna, only cook it for 1 minute per side; for medium, cook it for 2 minutes per side). Once the tuna is cooked to your desired doneness, quickly sear the edges of the steaks so that they are colored completely.

Serve immediately with the Asian Dipping Sauce. Store leftover tuna in an airtight container in the refrigerator for 1 to 2 days.

TURKEY, CRANBERRY, AND HONEY HERB CREAM CHEESE SANDWICH

After Thanksgiving, there is always the question of what to make with the leftovers. For me, it is this sandwich. What makes it so outstanding is the combination of sweet, herbed cream cheese, tart cranberry sauce, spicy arugula, and flavorful roast turkey. Your taste buds will be fully engaged by each mouthful. Enjoy with your favorite chips or salad. ❧ **MAKES 4 SANDWICHES**

1 cup cream cheese, at room temperature

¼ cup cranberry honey

1 tablespoon minced fresh parsley

1 tablespoon minced fresh thyme

1 green onion, minced

8 slices whole wheat or multigrain bread

¾–1 cup Cranberry Orange Sauce (page 174)

12 ounces Roasted Turkey Breast with Rhubarb Apple Glaze (page 122), sliced

1 cup arugula

In a small bowl, mix together the cream cheese, honey, parsley, thyme, and green onion until completely combined. Spread the honey cream cheese evenly on four slices of the bread. Spread the remaining four slices of bread with the Cranberry Orange Sauce.

Divide the turkey evenly among the bread slices spread with cream cheese. Add some arugula to each sandwich, then top with the other four slices of bread, cranberry sauce–side down. Cut the sandwiches in half diagonally, and serve.

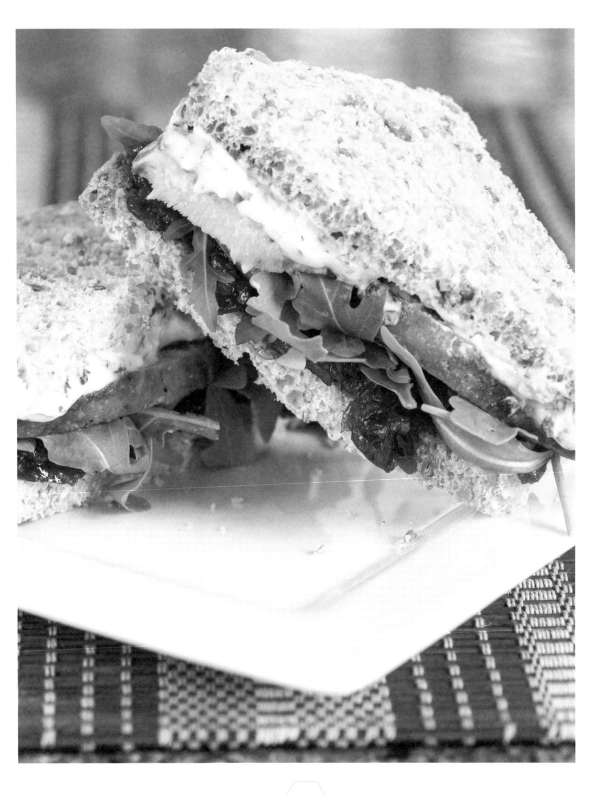

the asheville bee charmer cookbook

HONEY ROASTED PEAR, PARMESAN, AND PISTACHIO TART

When I worked at White Oak Gourmet, I made tarts every week, and this was one of my favorites. Who doesn't love cheese with fruits and nuts? We had adapted the crust from a recipe by gluten-free chef Elizabeth Barbone, and I have added dandelion honey, which enhances the flavor of the cheese in the crust. Roasting the pears with honey adds additional sweetness, but that's offset by the savory crust, the cheese, and the nuts. This is perfect for a light lunch or dinner with a glass of dry white wine. ❧ **MAKES 8 SERVINGS**

CRUST

1¼ cups gluten-free all-purpose flour

¼ cup tapioca starch

¾ cup shredded Parmigiano-Reggiano

½ teaspoon kosher salt

1 large egg

1 tablespoon dandelion honey

¼ cup cold unsalted butter, cut into small pieces

¼ cup very cold water

FILLING

2 tablespoons Corsican blossom honey

3 tablespoons olive oil

½ teaspoon kosher salt

¼ teaspoon freshly ground black pepper

3 Anjou pears, cut into ¼-inch cubes

3 large eggs

1 cup 2% milk

1 cup shredded Parmigiano-Reggiano

½ cup unsalted, roasted pistachios, shelled and roughly chopped

To make the crust, combine the gluten-free flour, tapioca starch, Parmigiano-Reggiano, salt, egg, dandelion honey, and butter in the bowl of a food processor. Pulse until everything is mixed together and the butter is broken into small pieces (it should look like lumpy wet sand). With the motor running, slowly add the water and process until the dough just comes together. Turn out the dough onto a work surface dusted lightly with gluten-free flour. Knead until the dough fully comes together and is no longer sticky. If the dough is too wet, add a bit more flour.

Press the dough evenly into an 11-inch tart pan with a removable bottom. Start on the bottom and then move your way up the sides. With the back of a ¼-cup measuring cup, starting from the center of the pan, press firmly in a circular pattern to even out the crust. Finish by pressing the cup around the bottom edge and against the sides of the tart pan. With a large knife, trim off any excess dough. Cover with plastic wrap and freeze for 1 hour.

Preheat the oven to 450°F. Line a baking sheet with parchment paper and set it aside.

To make the filling, whisk together the Corsican blossom honey, olive oil, salt, and pepper in a small bowl. Add the pears and mix well so that they are fully coated. Spread the pears out in a single layer on the prepared baking sheet and roast for 20 minutes, or until they are golden brown. Remove the baking sheet from the oven and let the pears cool.

Reduce the oven temperature to 350°F. Line another baking sheet with parchment paper.

Remove the crust from the freezer and place it on the prepared baking sheet. Bake for 15 minutes, or until the crust is just beginning to brown and no longer looks wet. Remove the crust from the oven, but do not turn off the oven.

In a small bowl, whisk together the eggs and milk until they are well incorporated and look like a custard base. Place the pears, Parmigiano-Reggiano, and pistachios in the tart crust and stir together gently. Pour the custard over the filling and press the ingredients down slightly.

Bake for 30 minutes, or until the tart is just set. Remove the tart from the oven and let it cool. Slice and serve at room temperature. Store leftover tart in an airtight container in the refrigerator for 4 to 5 days or in the freezer for up to 3 months.

PULLED PORK

I always think of pulled pork as one of those great dishes to have in the house on a Sunday afternoon, particularly during football season. It also works throughout the year for barbeques and picnics, or as an easy weeknight meal. The beauty of this recipe is that you make it in the slow cooker—you can turn it on in the morning and have a great meal waiting for you at dinnertime. With a slow cooker, your kitchen won't get hot while the pork is cooking, which is great in the summer. Serve on a bun for pulled pork sandwiches or on its own with a salad, slaw, or some chips. 🐝 **MAKES 8 SERVINGS**

1 tablespoon olive oil

1 tablespoon wildflower honey

1 tablespoon clover honey

2 tablespoons smoked paprika

1 tablespoon ancho chili powder

1 tablespoon ground cumin

1½ teaspoons ground coriander

1½ teaspoons freshly ground black pepper

2 teaspoons kosher salt

1 teaspoon red pepper flakes

1 (5–6 pound) pork shoulder roast

1 large yellow onion, cut into ¼-inch slices

5 cloves garlic, sliced

1½ cups water

2–3 cups Barbeque Sauce (page 178)

In a small bowl, whisk together the olive oil, wildflower honey, and clover honey. Add the paprika, chili powder, cumin, coriander, black pepper, salt, and red pepper flakes and whisk well. Rub the mixture all over the pork shoulder.

Place the onion, garlic, pork, and water in a slow cooker. Cover and cook on high for 3 hours. Reduce the heat to low and cook for another 5 to 6 hours, or until the pork begins to pull apart easily.

Transfer the pork shoulder to a bowl and let it rest for 10 to 15 minutes. Remove the garlic and onion from the slow cooker and skim off any fat from the cooking liquid.

While the pork is still warm, shred it with a fork, mixing in the cooking liquid. Add the Barbeque Sauce and stir well. Store leftover pulled pork in an airtight container in the refrigerator for up to 4 days or in the freezer for up to 3 months.

NOTE *If you don't have a slow cooker, you can place the pork in a roasting pan, cover it with parchment paper and then foil, so the pan is sealed tightly, and then cook it in a 300°F oven for 6 hours.*

APRICOT GLAZED CHICKEN KEBABS

After a lot of travel in Eastern Europe, the Middle East, and North Africa, I became a fan of eating meat dishes, particularly chicken and pork, cooked with fruit. The sweetness of the fruit, as long as it isn't cloying, complements the meat in a satisfying way. This dish works just as well with pork or turkey as it does with chicken. ❧ **MAKES 4 TO 5 SERVINGS**

¼ cup acacia honey

½ cup dried apricots, chopped into ¼-inch cubes

2 tablespoons tamari

1 tablespoon freshly squeezed lemon juice

2 cloves garlic, minced

½ teaspoon kosher salt

¼ teaspoon freshly ground black pepper

2 pounds boneless, skinless chicken breasts, cut into 1-inch cubes

To make the marinade, whisk together the honey, apricots, tamari, lemon juice, garlic, salt, and pepper in a small bowl. Place the chicken in a gallon-sized zip-top bag. Reserve ¼ cup of the marinade for grilling. Add the rest of the marinade to the bag and coat the chicken well. Seal the bag and let the chicken marinate at room temperature for 1 hour.

While the chicken is marinating, soak 15 to 20 (8-inch) wooden skewers in water for 10 to 15 minutes. Preheat a grill to medium high. Wipe off the excess marinade from the chicken and discard the marinade. Distribute the chicken evenly among the skewers.

Grill the kebabs for about 2 minutes per side, or until the chicken is fully cooked through. Remove the kebabs from the grill and baste them lightly with the reserved marinade. Serve immediately. Store leftover chicken in an airtight container in the refrigerator for up to 4 days.

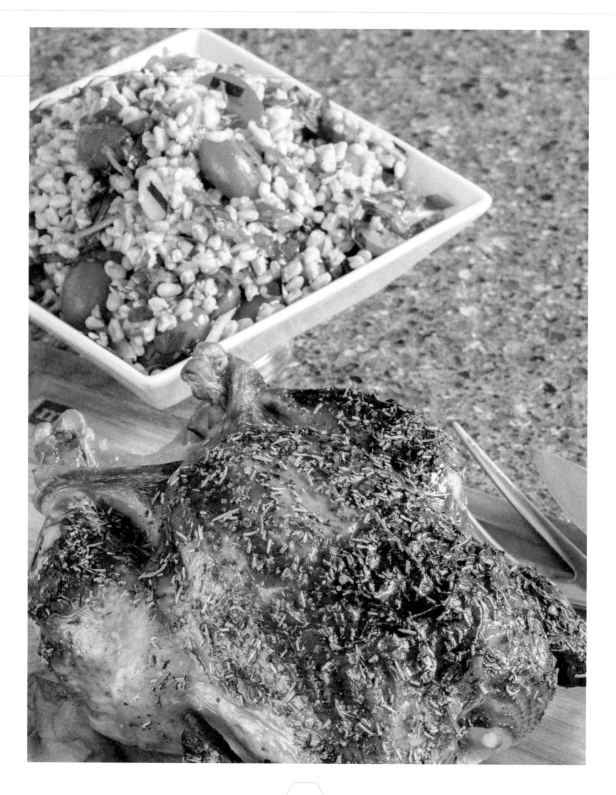

ROASTED HONEY GLAZED CHICKEN

This is my nod to rotisserie chicken. By cooking it on a rack, you allow air to flow around the chicken, which allows both the bottom and top to crisp. You can use fresh herbs, but I've found dried herbs provide a more intense flavor. The chicken gets very dark as it cooks because of the honey. If it looks like it's starting to burn, cover the chicken lightly with foil while it finishes cooking through. ✥ **MAKES 4 SERVINGS**

2 tablespoons olive oil

3 tablespoons Asheville Bee Charmer's Rosemary-Infused Honey, divided

1 teaspoon kosher salt

1 teaspoon dried rosemary

1 teaspoon dried thyme

½ teaspoon ground black pepper

1 lemon, cut in half crosswise

2 cloves garlic, roughly chopped

1 (3-pound) whole roasting chicken, rinsed and patted dry

Preheat the oven to 400°F. Line a baking sheet with aluminum foil, place a wire rack on top, and set it aside.

In a small bowl, whisk together the olive oil, honey, salt, rosemary, thyme, and pepper. Put the lemon and garlic inside the chicken cavity.

Rub the spiced oil and honey mixture all over the chicken and transfer the chicken to the wire rack on the prepared baking sheet. Roast the chicken for 30 minutes. Reduce the oven temperature to 350°F and continue roasting for about 1 hour, or until the chicken is golden brown and an instant-read thermometer inserted into the thickest part of the leg registers 165°F.

Remove the chicken from the oven, tent it with aluminum foil, and let it rest for at least 15 minutes before carving and serving. Store leftover chicken, bones removed, in an airtight container in the refrigerator for up to 4 days or in the freezer for up to 3 months.

Pictured at left, from top: Tuscan Farro (p. 142), Roasted Honey Glazed Chicken

PORK ADOBO

When I hear "pork adobo," I immediately think: Is it a Filipino adobo or a Mexican adobo? This is a Mexican version. Traditionally, the sauce calls for rehydrating dried chiles and then forming a paste or sauce with them. I use dried chili powder in this recipe because you can't always find the whole dried chiles, but you can always find chili powder. This recipe works just as well with chicken or beef. Try it served with rice or corn tortillas. ❧ **MAKES 6 TO 8 SERVINGS**

1 (3-pound) pork loin, cut into 1-inch cubes

1 large red onion, cut into ½-inch pieces (2 cups)

2 large red bell peppers, seeded and cut into ½-inch pieces (2 cups)

2 large green bell peppers, seeded and cut into ½-inch pieces (2 cups)

3 chipotle chiles in adobo sauce, cut into ¼-inch pieces

2 tablespoons minced garlic

2 teaspoons kosher salt

½ teaspoon freshly ground black pepper

1 tablespoon ancho chili powder

1 tablespoon ground coriander

1 tablespoon ground cumin

1 tablespoon dried oregano

2 bay leaves

2 tablespoons Asheville Bee Charmer's Smokin' Hot Honey (chipotle-infused honey)

2 tablespoons apple cider vinegar

Place all the ingredients in a slow cooker. Stir well so that everything is well coated with the spices. Cover and cook on low heat for 8 hours, or until the pork almost falls apart when pierced with a fork. Serve immediately. Store leftover pork in an airtight container in the refrigerator for up to 4 days or in the freezer for up to 3 months.

NOTE *If you don't have a slow cooker, you can place the pork mixture in a roasting pan, cover it with parchment paper and then foil, so that the pan is sealed tightly, and cook it in a 300°F oven for 3½ to 4 hours.*

BARBEQUE CHICKEN

This is the easiest barbeque chicken I have ever made. It's a one-pan dish; you sear it and then bake it in the same pan. By brushing the barbeque sauce on the chicken before it bakes, the sauce doesn't burn and the chicken remains moist. The honey is in the barbeque sauce, which has a sweet and spicy flavor. ❧ **MAKES 4 SERVINGS**

4 boneless, skinless chicken breasts (1¼–1½ pounds total)

¾ teaspoon kosher salt

¼ teaspoon freshly ground black pepper

1 tablespoon olive oil

½ cup Barbeque Sauce (page 178), plus more as desired

Preheat the oven to 350°F. Rinse the chicken breasts, pat them dry, and season them with the salt and pepper.

Heat the olive oil in a large, ovenproof sauté pan over medium-high heat until it's hot but not yet smoking. Add the chicken and sear it on one side for 3 minutes, or until it is golden brown. Flip the chicken and sear the other side for 3 minutes. Remove the pan from the heat and brush each chicken breast with 2 tablespoons of the Barbeque Sauce.

Transfer the pan to the oven and cook for 20 minutes, or until an instant-read thermometer inserted into the thickest part of a breast registers 165°F.

Serve with additional Barbeque Sauce, if desired. Store leftover chicken in an airtight container in the refrigerator for up to 4 days or in the freezer for up to 3 months.

MOROCCAN CHICKEN

This dish is inspired by the fantastic chicken tagines I've had throughout the years. I make mine in a slow cooker, as the cooking time lets the flavors meld and helps maintain the chicken's moisture. Try serving the chicken with Moroccan Couscous (page 137) and your favorite salad. ❧ **MAKES 6 TO 8 SERVINGS**

1 pound russet potatoes, cut into 1-inch cubes

1 tablespoon olive oil

8 boneless, skinless chicken thighs (about 1½–2 pounds total)

1 large yellow onion, cut into ¼-inch cubes (2 cups)

2 medium carrots, cut into ¼-inch cubes (1 cup)

2 large stalks celery, cut into ¼-inch cubes (¾ cup)

1 teaspoon kosher salt

½ teaspoon freshly ground black pepper

1 tablespoon smoked paprika

½ teaspoon garlic powder

1 teaspoon ground cumin

½ teaspoon ground coriander

½ teaspoon ground turmeric

1 teaspoon ground ginger

½ teaspoon ground cardamom

½ teaspoon ground allspice

1 teaspoon clover honey

1 teaspoon ginger-infused honey

1 tablespoon tomato powder or tomato paste

2 cups unsalted or low-sodium chicken stock

½ cup pitted dates, cut into ¼-inch cubes

½ cup sliced almonds

½ cup currants

1 large zucchini, cut into ½-inch cubes (2 cups)

Place the potatoes in a slow cooker.

In a large sauté pan, heat the oil over medium-high heat until it's hot but not smoking. Add the chicken and sear it for 3 minutes, or until it is golden brown. Flip the chicken and sear the other side for 3 minutes. Remove the chicken from the pan and set it on top of the potatoes in the slow cooker.

In the same sauté pan, combine the onion, carrots, and celery and sauté for 5 minutes, or until the vegetables have softened. Add the salt, pepper, paprika, garlic powder, cumin, coriander, turmeric, ginger, cardamom, allspice, clover honey, ginger honey, and tomato powder. Sauté for 1 minute, or until the spices become fragrant. Add the mixture to the slow cooker.

Pour the chicken stock into the slow cooker, then add the dates, almonds, currants, and zucchini. Gently stir to mix well. Cover the slow cooker and cook on low for 6 hours. Serve immediately. Store leftover chicken in an airtight container in the refrigerator for up to 4 days or in the freezer for up to 3 months.

NOTE *If you don't have a slow cooker, you can place the chicken mixture in a roasting pan, cover it with parchment paper and then foil, so that the pan is sealed tightly, and cook it in a 300°F oven for 3 to 4 hours.*

ROASTED PORK TENDERLOIN WITH APRICOT CHUTNEY

The chutney is what sets this dish apart. It is more oniony than traditional chutneys—I purposefully used dried onion to get a more concentrated flavor. It also uses Aleppo pepper, which makes it tangy. If you can't find Aleppo pepper, you can use red pepper flakes. If you have any leftover chutney, try using it to make baked Brie with fruit. ❧ **MAKES 4 SERVINGS**

1½ cups dried apricots, cut into ¼-inch cubes

¼ cup dried minced onion

2 tablespoons dried cranberries

2 tablespoons raisins

2 tablespoons basswood honey

2 tablespoons apple cider vinegar

1 teaspoon ground ginger

½ teaspoon dry mustard

1 teaspoon Aleppo pepper flakes

1¼ teaspoons kosher salt, divided

1½ cups water

2 tablespoons grapeseed oil

2 pounds pork tenderloin

½ teaspoon freshly ground black pepper

To make the chutney, in a medium saucepan set over medium-high heat, mix together the apricots, onion, cranberries, raisins, honey, vinegar, ginger, mustard, Aleppo pepper, ¼ teaspoon of the salt, and the water. Bring the mixture to a boil, then cover the pan, reduce the heat to low, and cook for 25 minutes, stirring every 10 minutes. If the mixture looks like it's drying out too much, add more water, ¼ cup at a time. Remove the pan from the heat and let the chutney cool to room temperature.

Preheat the oven to 400°F.

In a large ovenproof sauté pan, heat the grapeseed oil over medium-high heat until it's hot but not yet smoking. Sprinkle the pork with the remaining 1 teaspoon of salt and the black pepper, then add it to the pan. Sear the pork for 3 to 4 minutes per side (including the ends), or until it is nicely browned all over. Transfer the pan to the oven and cook for 10 minutes, or until an instant-read thermometer inserted into the thickest part of the meat registers 140°F.

Remove the pan from the oven and let the pork rest for 10 minutes. Slice the pork against the grain and serve with the chutney. Store leftover pork in an airtight container in the refrigerator for up to 4 days or in the freezer for up to 3 months. Store leftover chutney separately in an airtight container for up to 2 weeks.

ASIAN TURKEY LETTUCE CUPS

A couple of years ago, I had a personal chef client who wanted to eat carbohydrate-free, healthy, flavorful meals. As a result, I started making a lot of dishes in lettuce cups—from fajitas to Asian stir-fry. This is one of those recipes. It has loads of vegetables in it, but you can substitute based on your preferences. If you don't like ground turkey, use ground chicken, pork, or beef instead. **MAKES 3 SERVINGS**

¼ cup tamari

1 teaspoon sesame oil

1 tablespoon rice vinegar

1 tablespoon sambal oelek

1 tablespoon ginger-infused honey

1 tablespoon Asheville Bee Charmer's Firecracker Hot Honey

1 tablespoon mirin

2 tablespoons grapeseed oil

8 ounces ground turkey

1 tablespoon minced garlic

1 tablespoon minced fresh ginger

¼ medium red bell pepper, seeded and cut into ¼-inch cubes (¼ cup)

¼ medium green bell pepper, seeded and cut into ¼-inch cubes (¼ cup)

½ cup stemmed shiitake mushrooms, cut in half and sliced ¼ inch thick

½ cup sugar snap peas, sliced ¼ inch thick on the bias

2 green onions, sliced ¼ inch thick on the bias

12 leaves butter lettuce

3 tablespoons minced fresh cilantro

3 tablespoons toasted sesame seeds

In a measuring cup, whisk together the tamari, sesame oil, vinegar, sambal oelek, ginger honey, Firecracker Hot Honey, and mirin. Set aside.

In a large sauté pan set over medium-high heat, heat the grapeseed oil until it's hot but not yet smoking. Add the ground turkey, garlic, and ginger, breaking up the turkey with a wooden spoon. Cook for about 5 minutes, until the turkey is slightly browned. Add the red and green bell peppers and sauté for 1 minute. Add the mushrooms, snap peas, and green onions and sauté for 1 minute. Add the honey mixture and cook for about 5 minutes, until almost all the liquid is absorbed. Remove the pan from the heat.

Divide the turkey mixture among the 12 butter lettuce leaves. Garnish each lettuce cup evenly with the cilantro and sesame seeds. Place four lettuce cups on each plate and serve immediately. Store leftover filling in an airtight container in the refrigerator for up to 4 days.

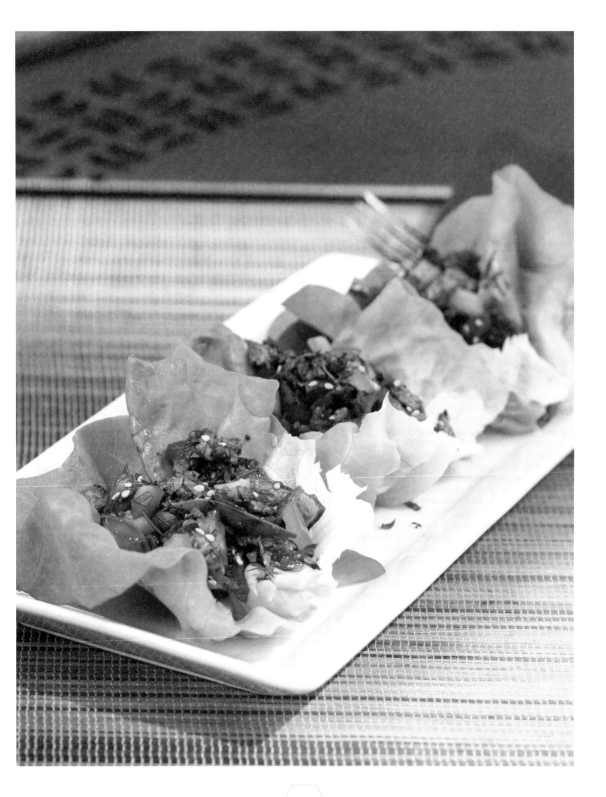

KOREAN FLANK STEAK

Chicago has a lot of great restaurants serving Korean barbeque. The steak is always tender and flavorful, with a slightly sweet soy, ginger, garlic, and pepper marinade. This is my take on those flavors. It certainly isn't a traditional blend of ingredients, but it mimics the flavor well. ❧ **MAKES 2 TO 3 SERVINGS**

¼ cup tamari

¼ cup buckwheat honey

2 tablespoons sake

1 tablespoon tahini

1 tablespoon sambal oelek

2 tablespoons Worcestershire sauce

6 cloves garlic, minced

2 green onions, minced

1 teaspoon freshly ground black pepper

1 pound flank steak

To make the marinade, whisk together the tamari, honey, sake, tahini, sambal oelek, Worcestershire sauce, garlic, green onions, and black pepper in a small bowl. Place the steak in a gallon-sized zip-top bag. Add the marinade and coat the steak well. Seal the bag and let the steak marinate at room temperature for 1 hour.

Heat a grill to medium high. Wipe off the excess marinade from the steak and discard the marinade. Grill the steak for 7 to 8 minutes per side (for medium rare), or until it's cooked to your liking.

Transfer the steak to a plate, tent it with foil, and let it rest for at least 10 minutes. Cut the steak against the grain and serve immediately. Store leftover meat in an airtight container in the refrigerator for up to 4 days or in the freezer for up to 3 months.

SWEET AND SOUR TOFU NOODLES

I have always been intrigued by the complexity of flavors in Thai dishes. The balance of sweet, sour, salty, bitter, and spicy can be magical. Other than fish sauce, I don't use traditional Thai ingredients, but these noodles are an homage to one of the greatest cuisines in the world.

❧ MAKES 4 SERVINGS

1 tablespoon yellow miso paste

¼ cup fish sauce

½ cup rice wine vinegar

1 cup carrot honey

3 tablespoons tomato paste

1 teaspoon chili powder

1 teaspoon freshly grated lime zest

¼ cup tamari

¼ cup water

1 (16-ounce) box dried flat rice noodles

¼ cup grapeseed oil

2 teaspoons minced garlic

¼ cup minced shallot

4 large eggs, beaten

1 cup extra-firm tofu, cut into ¼-inch cubes

2 cups bean sprouts

2 green onions, minced

2 tablespoons minced fresh cilantro (leaves and stems)

1 cup salted, roasted peanuts, roughly chopped

In a small bowl, whisk together the miso, fish sauce, rice wine vinegar, honey, tomato paste, chili powder, lime zest, tamari, and water until well incorporated. Set aside.

In a medium bowl, soak the rice noodles in enough hot water (about 90°F) to cover for 10 minutes. Drain. Squeeze out any excess liquid and set the noodles aside.

In a wok or large sauté pan over medium-high heat, heat the grapeseed oil until it's hot but not yet smoking. Add the garlic and shallot and cook for 1 to 2 minutes, or until golden brown. Add the soaked noodles and stir-fry until they just start to crisp, about 5 to 7 minutes.

Add the honey mixture and cook until almost all the liquid is gone, about 5 minutes. Add the eggs and cook, stirring constantly, until they have scrambled. Add the tofu and cook for 2 minutes, or until lightly browned. Remove the pan from the heat and stir in the bean sprouts, green onions, cilantro, and peanuts. Serve immediately. Store leftover noodles in an airtight container in the refrigerator for up to 4 days.

GINGER LIME SHRIMP

This dish uses pan-Asian ingredients with an emphasis on spicy ginger and acidic lime. I marinate and cook the shrimp in their shells because it helps them stay plump and juicy. Don't marinate them for much longer than an hour because, given their small size, they can easily become over seasoned. ❧ **MAKES 4 SERVINGS**

2 tablespoons minced fresh ginger	**2 tablespoons freshly squeezed lime juice**
2 tablespoons tamari	**2 green onions, minced**
1 tablespoon ginger-infused honey	**1½ pounds (20–25 count) shrimp, shells on**
2 tablespoons sake	**2 tablespoons grapeseed oil**

To make the marinade, whisk together the ginger, tamari, ginger honey, sake, lime juice, and green onions in a small bowl. Devein the shrimp and place them in a gallon-sized zip-top bag. Add the marinade, seal the bag, and shake until the shrimp are well coated. Let the shrimp marinate at room temperature for 1 hour.

Remove the shrimp from the marinade and discard the marinade.

Heat the oil in a large sauté pan over high heat until it's hot but not yet smoking. Add the shrimp and cook for 2 to 3 minutes, or until their bottoms are pink. Flip the shrimp and cook for 2 minutes, or until the other side is pink and the shrimp have just cooked through.

Transfer the shrimp to a heatproof bowl and cover with plastic wrap. Let the shrimp steam for 10 to 15 minutes. Remove the shells from the shrimp and serve immediately. Store leftover shrimp in an airtight container in the refrigerator for 1 to 2 days.

DUCK À L'ORANGE

You can't get a more traditional French dish than duck à l'orange. There is something really special about the flavor combination of duck and orange. However, this is not a traditional way to make the duck, and I have eliminated a number of steps in making the sauce. What you end up with is a sauce that can hold its own against a more traditional preparation.

🐝 **MAKES 2 SERVINGS**

2 duck breasts (about 1 pound total)

1 teaspoon kosher salt, plus more to taste

½ teaspoon freshly ground black pepper, plus more to taste

½ cup freshly squeezed orange juice

¼ cup dry white wine

2 teaspoons orange blossom honey

½ cup unsalted or low-sodium chicken stock

¼ teaspoon dried thyme

1 orange, peeled and segmented

Wash and dry the duck. Using a small, sharp knife, score the skin of the duck by making shallow incisions in a crosshatch pattern across the entire breast. Make sure not to cut into the flesh of the duck. Season the duck with the salt and pepper.

Place the duck skin-side down in a large, cold sauté pan. Place a second sauté pan on top of the duck and weight it down with a metal can. Cook the duck over medium heat for 8 to 10 minutes, until all the fat is rendered and the skin is brown and crispy. Remove the weight and the second pan. Drain off the extra fat and discard it or reserve it for another use.

Increase the heat to medium high and flip the duck. Cook for 6 minutes, or until an instant-read thermometer inserted into the thickest part of a breast registers 135°F. Transfer the duck to a warm plate, tent it with foil, and let it rest while you make the sauce.

To make the sauce, drain any remaining fat from the sauté pan and return it to medium-high heat. Add the orange juice and wine and bring the liquid to a boil. Let it boil for 3 to 4 minutes, or until it has reduced to 1 to 2 tablespoons of liquid.

Whisk in the honey, chicken stock, and thyme. Bring the liquid to a boil and reduce until thickened, about 3 to 4 minutes. If any juices have pooled around the resting duck, stir them into the sauce. Gently stir in the orange segments. Taste and season with the salt and pepper, if necessary.

Slice the duck on the bias. Divide the sauce between two plates and place one duck breast on each plate. Serve immediately. Store leftover duck in an airtight container in the refrigerator for up to 4 days or in the freezer for up to 3 months.

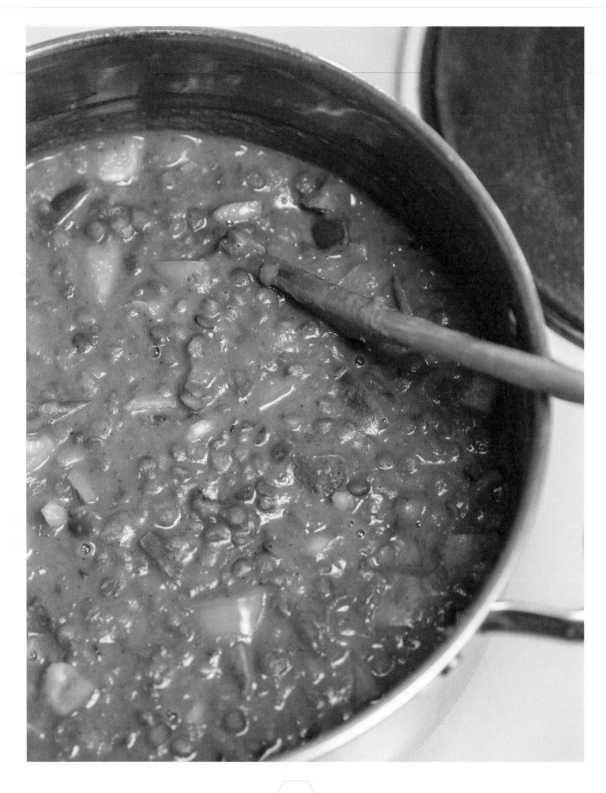

LENTIL AND SWEET POTATO STEW

I used to eat a lot of groundnut stew when I traveled in West Africa. This dish reminds me of those times, despite the lack of groundnuts (peanuts) in the stew. It's a hearty, protein-loaded vegetarian dish with a mellow curry flavor. Eat this stew on its own, with some rice, or over Carrot Freekeh (page 133). ❧ **MAKES 6 SERVINGS**

2 tablespoons olive oil

1 yellow bell pepper, seeded and chopped into ¼-inch cubes

1 green bell pepper, seeded and chopped into ¼-inch cubes

2 medium sweet potatoes, peeled and chopped into ¼-inch cubes (2–3 cups)

2 tablespoons minced fresh ginger

2 tablespoons Madras curry powder

1 teaspoon kosher salt

1 (15-ounce) can coconut milk

1 (15-ounce) can diced tomatoes

2 cups unsalted or low-sodium vegetable stock

1 tablespoon freshly squeezed lemon juice

2 tablespoons clover honey

3 cups cooked brown lentils

In a 6-quart stockpot set over medium-high heat, heat the oil until it's hot but not yet smoking. Add the yellow and green bell peppers and sauté until they are soft, about 5 minutes. Add the sweet potatoes and sauté for 5 minutes. Stir in the ginger, curry powder, and salt and sauté for 1 minute, or until fragrant. Stir in the coconut milk, diced tomatoes (including juices), vegetable stock, lemon juice, honey, and lentils. Bring the liquid to a boil, then cover the pot, reduce the heat to low, and simmer for 30 minutes, or until the sweet potatoes are fully cooked through and soft.

Serve immediately with your favorite grain. Store leftover stew in an airtight container in the refrigerator for up to 5 days or in the freezer for up to 6 months.

ROASTED TURKEY BREAST WITH RHUBARB APPLE GLAZE

Last winter, I cleaned out my freezer and found a bag of frozen rhubarb from the previous spring harvest. I wanted to use it in a sauce, but I didn't have any fresh or frozen strawberries, so I used some apples I had lying around. The sauce was wonderful, and I ended up using some of it as a glaze on a turkey breast. It's a unique alternative to eating turkey with cranberry sauce. ✤ **MAKES 8 SERVINGS**

1 (4½-pound) fresh bone-in, skin-on turkey breast

1 tablespoon olive oil

¾ teaspoon kosher salt

¼ teaspoon freshly ground black pepper

½ cup Rhubarb Apple Sauce (page 178), plus more for serving

Preheat the oven to 400°F. Line a baking sheet with aluminum foil, place a wire rack on top, and set it aside.

Rinse the turkey and pat it dry. Rub the olive oil all over the turkey and season with the salt and pepper. Place the turkey skin-side up on the rack on the prepared baking sheet.

Place the turkey in the oven and roast for 30 minutes, then remove it from the oven and reduce the oven temperature to 350°F. Brush ¼ cup of the Rhubarb Apple Sauce on the turkey, return the turkey to the oven, and roast for 40 more minutes. Remove the turkey again, brush it with the remaining ¼ cup of Rhubarb Apple Sauce, and return it to the oven for another 35 to 40 minutes, or until an instant-read thermometer inserted into the thickest part of the breast registers 165°F.

Turn on the broiler and broil the turkey breast for 1 to 2 minutes, or until the glaze just begins to caramelize and brown. Remove the turkey from the oven, tent it with foil, and let it rest for at least 15 minutes before slicing. Serve with warmed Rhubarb Apple Sauce. Store leftover turkey, bones removed, in an airtight container in the refrigerator for up to 4 days or in the freezer for up to 3 months.

ASIAN EDAMAME BURGERS

There is a small burger chain in Chicago called Tom & Eddie's. Their delicious edamame burger inspired this one. I've made the burger gluten free by using buckwheat as one of the binding ingredients. Despite the number of ingredients, this is easy to put together. After the burgers are baked, you can cool and freeze the leftovers. Just reheat the burgers in the oven as you need them. ❧ **MAKES 8 BURGERS**

⅔ cup water

⅓ cup uncooked whole-grain buckwheat groats

1 teaspoon kosher salt

1 (16-ounce) package frozen shelled edamame, thawed

3 tablespoons peeled, sliced fresh ginger

1 tablespoon ginger-infused honey

1 cup grated carrot

3 large eggs

3 tablespoons freshly squeezed lemon juice

2 tablespoons mirin

3 tablespoons sambal oelek

2 tablespoons tamari

1½ cups gluten-free panko breadcrumbs

8 gluten-free hamburger buns

½ cup tahini

2 cups Hearty Greens Slaw (page 85)

Preheat the oven to 375°F. Line a baking sheet with parchment paper and grease it with non-stick cooking spray.

Bring the water to a boil in a medium saucepan set over medium-high heat. Add the buckwheat and salt. Bring to a boil. Cover the pan, reduce the heat to low, and simmer for 10 minutes. Remove the pan from the heat, keeping the lid on, and let the buckwheat steam for 15 minutes.

In the bowl of a food processor, combine the edamame, ginger, and ginger honey. Process for 3 to 5 minutes, stopping to scrape down the sides of the bowl every 1 to 2 minutes, until the mixture is finely chopped.

Transfer the mixture to a large bowl. Add the cooked buckwheat, carrot, eggs, lemon juice, mirin, sambal oelek, tamari, and breadcrumbs. Wearing latex gloves, use your hands to mix everything together until it's completely incorporated (if you don't want to mix with your hands, use a rubber spatula). Cover the bowl and let the mixture rest for 10 minutes at room temperature.

Portion out ¾ cup of the burger mixture and form it into a patty. Place it on the prepared baking sheet. Repeat this process until all of the mixture has been used. Lightly spray the patties with nonstick cooking spray and transfer them to the oven.

Bake the patties for 10 minutes, then flip them and bake for another 15 minutes, or until they are golden brown. Remove the patties from the oven.

Spread the tahini evenly on the bottom half of each bun. Add the burgers, top each with ¼ cup of the Hearty Greens Slaw, and then add the top half of each bun. Serve immediately. Store leftover patties in an airtight container in the refrigerator for up to 5 days.

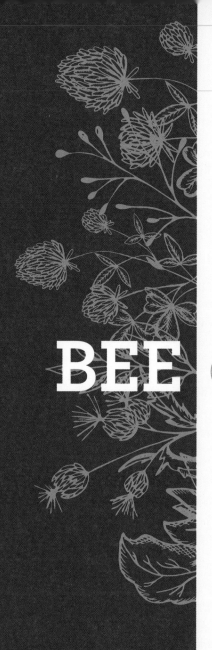

BEE Complementary

CHAPTER 5

Sides

HONEY ROASTED BRUSSELS SPROUTS

Honey and Brussels sprouts? Absolutely! After living in London for five years, I used to eat Brussels sprouts that had been boiled and sautéed in butter with chestnuts. Then I tried them roasted and was blown away by how tasty they were. Roasting them with honey and oil kicks things up another notch. They are like candy—you won't be able to stop eating them.

MAKES 4 SERVINGS

1 pound Brussels sprouts
¼ cup olive oil
2 tablespoons sourwood honey

½ teaspoon kosher salt
¼ teaspoon freshly ground black pepper

Preheat the oven to 450°F. Line a baking sheet with parchment paper or aluminum foil and set it aside.

Thoroughly wash the Brussels sprouts, trim the bottoms, and slice them in half lengthwise.

Place the sprouts in a bowl. Add the oil and sourwood honey. Season with the salt and pepper and mix until the sprouts are thoroughly coated. Transfer the sprouts, cut-side down, to the prepared baking sheet.

Roast for 12 to 13 minutes. They should be getting browned at this point. Turn them over and roast for another 12 to 13 minutes, or until they are fork tender. Remove the Brussels sprouts from the oven and serve immediately. Store leftover Brussels sprouts in an airtight container in the refrigerator for up to 4 days.

BOLIVIAN BAKED BUCKWHEAT

I originally tried a variation of this on a trip to Bolivia, but it was made with quinoa. I like quinoa, but I find it used in an overabundance of recipes. Buckwheat, an underutilized grain with many health benefits, has a nuttier, heartier flavor than quinoa that works well with the tomatoes, spices, and cheese in this recipe. ✷ **MAKES 8 TO 10 SERVINGS**

3 cups water

1½ cups uncooked whole-grain buckwheat groats

2 teaspoons kosher salt, divided

1 tablespoon grapeseed oil

1 medium yellow onion, cut into ¼-inch cubes

1 (14.5-ounce) can diced tomatoes

2 tablespoons minced fresh flat-leaf parsley

1 teaspoon dried oregano

1 teaspoon buckwheat honey

½ teaspoon ground allspice

½ teaspoon freshly ground black pepper

1 teaspoon Tabasco sauce

1 cup unsalted or low-sodium vegetable stock

½ cup gluten-free all-purpose flour

3 large eggs

¾ cup whole or 2% milk

8 ounces sharp white cheddar, shredded

Preheat the oven to 375°F. Grease a 10-inch round baking dish (one with sides at least 3 inches high works best) with nonstick cooking spray.

In a medium saucepan over medium-high heat, bring the water to a boil. Add the buckwheat and 1 teaspoon of the salt. Bring the water back to a boil, then cover the pan, reduce the heat to low, and simmer for 10 minutes. Remove the pan from the heat, keeping the lid on, and let the buckwheat steam for 15 minutes. Spread the steamed buckwheat out on a baking sheet and let it cool.

In a large sauté pan, heat the oil over medium-high heat until it's hot but not yet smoking. Add the onion and cook for 5 to 8 minutes, or until it has softened and starts to brown on the edges. Add the tomatoes, parsley, oregano, honey, allspice, black pepper, Tabasco sauce, and the remaining 1 teaspoon of salt. Cook for 5 minutes, stirring constantly. Add the vegetable stock and simmer for 10 minutes.

In a large bowl, toss the cooled buckwheat with the flour. In a measuring cup, whisk together the eggs and milk. Add the egg mixture to the buckwheat and stir. Add the tomato mixture and half of the cheese. Stir well, pour the mixture into the prepared pan, and sprinkle the remaining cheese on top.

Bake for 40 to 45 minutes, or until the top is nicely browned. Remove the pan from the oven and let the casserole rest for 5 to 10 minutes before serving. Store leftovers in an airtight container in the refrigerator for up to 5 days.

HONEY ROASTED ROOT VEGETABLES

Roasting root vegetables brings out their natural sweetness, as it causes the sugar in the vegetables to caramelize. The carrot honey in this recipe makes those flavors more intense. These vegetables are perfect on their own, but if you have leftovers, they are great thrown into a soup or tossed with some pasta and olive oil. ❦ **MAKES 4 SERVINGS**

6 cups cubed mixed root vegetables (about ½ inch in size)

¼ cup olive oil

2 tablespoons carrot honey

½ teaspoon kosher salt

¼ teaspoon freshly ground black pepper

Preheat the oven to 450°F. Line a baking sheet with parchment paper and set it aside.

Place the root vegetables in a large bowl. In a small bowl, whisk together the oil and carrot honey. Add the honey mixture to the vegetables. Season with the salt and pepper and toss to coat evenly.

Transfer the vegetables to the prepared baking sheet and spread them out evenly. Place the baking sheet in the oven and roast the vegetables for 15 minutes, then remove the baking sheet from the oven, stir the vegetables, and return them to the oven for another 10 minutes, or until the vegetables are browned and fork tender. Remove the vegetables from the oven and serve immediately. Store leftover root vegetables in an airtight container in the refrigerator for up to 4 days.

NOTE *Use any combination of root vegetables you like: carrot, celery root, parsnip, turnip, rutabaga, sweet potato, butternut squash, acorn squash, kabocha squash, or beet.*

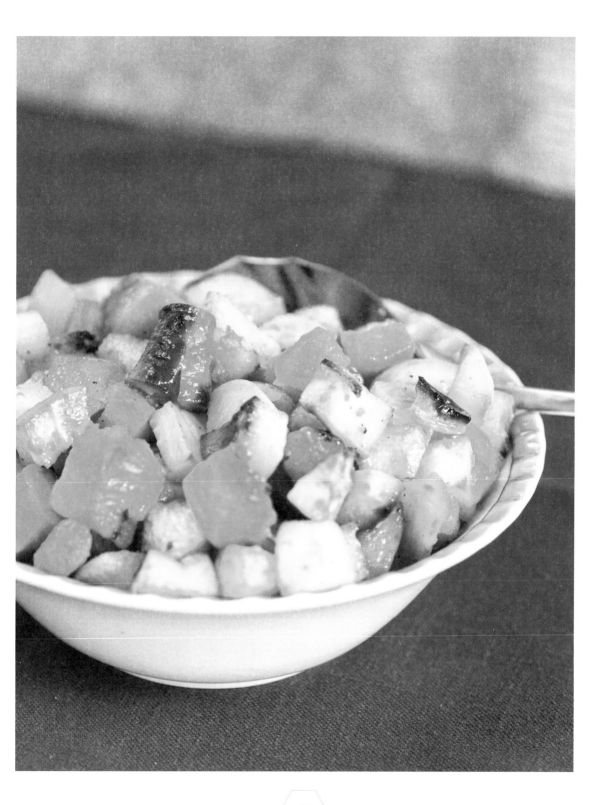

the asheville bee charmer cookbook

SWEET AND SPICY CABBAGE AND BEETS

 GF V

This recipe has its roots in French braised cabbage. As the cabbage cooks, it becomes sweeter. The beet and cranberry juice add flavor and intensify the dish's color, while the jalapeños and Ghost Pepper Honey add spice. ꙮ **MAKES 4 TO 5 SERVINGS**

2 tablespoons olive oil

½ large red onion, cut into ⅛-inch slices (about 1 cup)

1 large red beet, peeled and cut into ¼-inch cubes (about 2 cups)

2 jalapeños, seeded, deveined, and finely chopped

1 large clove garlic, minced

½ head small red cabbage, quartered, cored, and sliced ¼ inch thick

1 teaspoon kosher salt

½ teaspoon dried thyme

1 tablespoon blueberry honey

1 tablespoon Asheville Bee Charmer's Ghost Pepper Honey

1½ cups unsweetened cranberry juice

1 tablespoon unsalted butter

In a medium saucepan, heat the olive oil over medium-high heat until it's hot but not yet smoking. Add the onion, beet, jalapeños, and garlic and cook, stirring occasionally, for 8 to 10 minutes, until the vegetables have softened.

Add the cabbage, salt, thyme, blueberry honey, Ghost Pepper Honey, and cranberry juice. Bring the liquid to a boil, then cover the pan, reduce the heat to low, and simmer for 1 hour, or until the beets and cabbage are soft. Check the cabbage periodically to make sure it hasn't dried out. If need be, add water, ¼ cup at a time.

Stir in the butter and serve immediately. Store leftovers in an airtight container in the refrigerator for 4 to 5 days.

EGGPLANT PARMESAN STACKS

My test of an Italian restaurant is whether it has a good eggplant parmesan. This healthier spin on this classic dish is gluten free and stacked. The ingredients are traditional, but instead of being fried and baked, they are roasted and baked. Despite this difference, these stacks are just as flavorful as the traditional dish. ❧ **MAKES 4 TO 5 SERVINGS**

¼ cup olive oil

2 tablespoons balsamic vinegar

2 tablespoons dandelion honey

3 small eggplants (about 1¼ pounds total), cut into 30 (½-inch-thick) slices

1 teaspoon kosher salt, divided

½ teaspoon freshly ground black pepper, divided

4 vine-ripened tomatoes, cut into 20 (¼-inch-thick) slices

1 (1-pound) log fresh mozzarella, cut into 20 slices

30 fresh basil leaves, cut into chiffonade

½ cup + 2 tablespoons shredded Parmigiano-Reggiano

Preheat the oven to 400°F. Line two baking sheets with parchment paper and set them aside.

In a small bowl, whisk together the olive oil, balsamic vinegar, and honey. Place the eggplant slices on the prepared baking sheets. Brush the eggplant with some of the honey mixture and reserve the rest. Season with about half of the salt and pepper. Bake for 10 minutes, until just starting to brown.

Remove the baking sheets from the oven and flip the eggplant slices. Add the tomatoes to one of the baking sheets. Brush the eggplant and tomatoes with the rest of the honey mixture. Season with the remaining half of the salt and pepper. Bake for another 10 minutes, until the eggplant is just starting to brown. Remove the baking sheets from the oven. Slide the eggplant and tomatoes, with their parchment paper, off the baking sheet and onto a wire rack; let the vegetables cool slightly.

Reduce the oven temperature to 350°F. Place fresh parchment paper on one of the baking sheets.

To assemble the stacks, lay 10 slices of eggplant on the prepared baking sheet. Place a slice of tomato on top of each eggplant slice. Place a slice of mozzarella on top of each tomato slice. Sprinkle 1 teaspoon of Parmigiano-Reggiano on top and scatter on some basil leaves. Repeat the layering one more time. Finish each stack with a slice of eggplant topped with 1 teaspoon of Parmigiano-Reggiano. Each stack should have three slices of eggplant, two slices of tomato, two slices of mozzarella, two sprinkles of basil, and 3 teaspoons of Parmigiano-Reggiano.

Bake for 5 minutes, or until the mozzarella begins to melt slightly. Remove the baking sheet from the oven and sprinkle the stacks with any remaining basil. Serve immediately or at room temperature. Store leftover stacks in an airtight container in the refrigerator for up to 4 days.

CAPONATA

The trick to making a good caponata is to cook each vegetable separately. Most caponata recipes call for the vegetables to be mixed together and cooked in a pot until they are like a stew. My version is a lot chunkier and less saucy than a typical caponata. It's delicious with a crusty baguette. Leftovers can be tossed with pasta or used as an omelet filling. ✻ **MAKES 4 CUPS**

2 cups water

2 stalks celery, cut into ½-inch cubes

¼ cup olive oil, divided

¼ large red onion, chopped into ½-inch cubes (½ cup)

2 cloves garlic, minced

1 teaspoon kosher salt, divided

½ teaspoon freshly ground black pepper, divided

1 large eggplant, peeled and cut into ½-inch cubes

¼ cup pitted green olives, chopped

¼ cup niçoise olives, chopped

3 tablespoons capers, rinsed

1 (15-ounce) can diced tomatoes, drained

2 tablespoons red wine vinegar

3 tablespoons acacia honey

In a small saucepan set over high heat, bring the water to a boil. Add the celery and blanch it for 2 minutes. Remove the pan from the heat, drain the celery, and set it aside.

Heat 1 tablespoon of the oil in a large sauté pan over medium-high heat until it's hot but not yet smoking. Add the onion, garlic, ¼ teaspoon of the salt, and ⅛ teaspoon of the pepper and sauté for about 5 minutes, until the onion is soft and slightly browned. Spoon the onion into a large bowl and set it aside.

Return the sauté pan to medium-high heat and add 1 tablespoon of the oil. When the oil is hot, add the blanched celery and season with ¼ teaspoon of the salt and ⅛ teaspoon of the pepper. Sauté for about 7 minutes, until the celery is fork tender and slightly browned. Remove the pan from the heat and add the celery to the onions.

Return the sauté pan to medium-high heat and add the remaining 2 tablespoons of oil. When the oil is hot, add the eggplant and season with the remaining ½ teaspoon of salt and the remaining ¼ teaspoon of pepper. Sauté for 8 to 10 minutes, or until the eggplant is cooked through and slightly browned. Remove the pan from the heat and add the eggplant to the celery and onions. Add the green and niçoise olives, capers, and diced tomatoes to the vegetables. Stir well.

In a small bowl, whisk together the vinegar and honey. Add the honey mixture to the vegetables and stir well so that everything is evenly coated. Serve at room temperature. Store leftover caponata in an airtight container in the refrigerator for 4 to 5 days.

CARROT FREEKEH

Freekeh, a protein-loaded ancient grain, is wheat that has been harvested early, while the grains are still tender and green. The kernels are then roasted, dried, and rubbed. It has a chewy texture and a slightly nutty flavor—a great grain to add to your repertoire. Cooking grains with stock or flavored liquid, rather than plain water, infuses them with additional seasoning. In this dish, adding carrot juice not only does that, but it will also turn your cooked freekeh orange, a colorful and fun addition to any plate! Try this with a simply prepared protein or Lentil and Sweet Potato Stew (page 121). ❧ **MAKES ABOUT 5 CUPS**

1 tablespoon olive oil

¼ large yellow onion, cut into ¼-inch cubes (½ cup)

1 stalk celery, cut into ¼-inch cubes (½ cup)

1 cup uncooked freekeh

2½ cups carrot juice

1 tablespoon carrot honey

½ teaspoon kosher salt

¼ teaspoon freshly ground black pepper

Heat the oil in a medium saucepan over medium heat until it's hot but not yet smoking. Add the onion and celery and sweat them, stirring occasionally, for 5 to 8 minutes, or until they are softened and the onion is translucent. Add the freekeh to the pan and cook for about 3 minutes, stirring constantly, until the grains are slightly toasted. Add the carrot juice, honey, salt, and pepper and stir well.

Bring the mixture to a boil, then cover the pan, reduce the heat to low, and simmer for 45 to 55 minutes, until almost all the liquid has been absorbed. Remove the pan from the heat, keeping the lid on, and let the freekeh steam for 10 minutes. Serve warm. Store leftover freekeh in an airtight container in the refrigerator for 4 to 5 days.

ROASTED SPAGHETTI SQUASH
WITH HERBS

Spaghetti squash is a satisfying alternative to pasta. You can cook it in a microwave, but the flavor is enhanced when you roast it. A simple way to prepare it is to throw some herbs and shredded Parmigiano-Reggiano on it. You can also serve it with your favorite tomato or pesto sauce. **MAKES 6 SERVINGS**

2 tablespoons olive oil

1 tablespoon Corsican blossom honey

1 large spaghetti squash, halved lengthwise and seeded

1 teaspoon kosher salt, plus more to taste

½ teaspoon freshly ground black pepper, plus more to taste

¼ cup minced fresh thyme

½ cup minced fresh flat-leaf parsley

¼ cup minced green onion

½ cup unsalted, toasted hazelnuts, roughly chopped

1 cup shredded Parmigiano-Reggiano

Preheat the oven to 400°F. Line a baking sheet with parchment paper and set it aside.

In a small bowl, whisk together the oil and honey. Brush the honey mixture on the cut sides of the spaghetti squash. Season with the salt and pepper. Place the squash cut-side down on the prepared baking sheet.

Roast the squash for 45 minutes, or until it is soft and you can easily pierce the skin with a knife. Remove the squash from the oven and let it cool slightly. With a fork, carefully scrape the flesh in long strands into a medium bowl. Add the thyme, parsley, green onion, and hazelnuts and toss to incorporate completely. Taste and season with additional salt and pepper, if needed.

Divide the squash evenly among six plates. Sprinkle with the Parmigiano-Reggiano and serve immediately. Store leftovers in an airtight container in the refrigerator for up to 4 days.

MILK AND HONEY DINNER ROLLS

These dinner rolls are almost reminiscent of Hawaiian rolls or challah. They have a sweet quality to them because of the honey, but they are also rich because of the milk. Once these are baked and cooled, I usually freeze half of them for later. Simply reheat them in the oven to warm them up and serve. They are nice to have alongside dinner, to use to make a small sandwich, or as a snack with some cheese or a big pat of butter. ❧ **MAKES 15 ROLLS**

1½ teaspoons active dry yeast

1 cup 2% milk, warmed to about 90°F

3 cups all-purpose flour

3 tablespoons wildflower honey

1½ teaspoons kosher salt

2 large eggs, divided

5 tablespoons unsalted butter

1 tablespoon water

In the bowl of a stand mixer fitted with the dough hook, mix together the yeast and milk. Let the mixture stand for about 5 minutes, or until it foams.

Add the flour, honey, salt, 1 of the eggs, and the butter. Mix on low speed for 4 minutes, or until well combined. Increase the speed to medium and continue mixing for another 10 minutes, or until the dough is smooth and elastic.

Grease a large bowl lightly with grapeseed oil. Transfer the dough to the prepared bowl, cover it with plastic wrap, and let the dough rise in an unheated oven for 1 hour, or until it has doubled in size.

Line two baking sheets with parchment paper and set them aside.

Divide the dough into 15 (2-ounce) balls. Roll one ball into a 9-inch rope. Wrap the rope around your fingers. Take one end over the top of the rope and pull it through the hole in the center. Lightly pinch the other end of the rope to the bottom of the roll. It should look like a small round with a button in the center. Repeat the process with the remaining dough balls. Transfer the rolls to the prepared baking sheets, spacing them about 2 inches apart. Let the rolls rise, uncovered, in an unheated oven for 1 hour.

Remove the rolls from the oven and preheat it to 350°F. To make an egg wash, whisk the remaining egg and the water together. Lightly brush the rolls with the egg wash.

Bake for 25 to 30 minutes, or until the rolls are golden brown and an instant-read thermometer inserted into the center of a roll registers 190°F. Remove the rolls from the oven and serve slightly warm. Store leftover rolls in an airtight container at room temperature for 1 to 2 days.

Pictured on p. 98

HONEY GLAZED CARROTS

If you want to get your kids, big or small, to eat carrots, there is no better way than to cook them with butter and honey. This is a very traditional French preparation for carrots, and it is simply delicious. I won't lie, I prefer to eat raw carrots rather than cooked carrots, but I never want to share when I make these. ✿ **MAKES 4 SERVINGS**

4 medium carrots, peeled and sliced ¼ inch thick on the bias (2 cups)

¼ teaspoon kosher salt

⅛ teaspoon freshly ground black pepper

½ teaspoon carrot honey

¼ cup water

2 tablespoons unsalted butter

1 tablespoon chopped fresh flat-leaf parsley, for garnish

Cut a piece of parchment paper into a round that fits inside a medium saucepan. Butter one side of it and set it aside.

In a medium saucepan, combine the carrots, salt, pepper, honey, water, and butter. Cover the mixture with the parchment, buttered-side down, and place the pan over medium-high heat. Cook for 10 minutes, shaking the saucepan every couple of minutes, until the liquid has evaporated, and the carrots are tender and appear lightly glazed.

Remove the pan from the heat, garnish with the parsley, and serve. Store leftover carrots in an airtight container in the refrigerator for up to 4 days.

MOROCCAN COUSCOUS

Couscous needs to be made with flavored cooking liquid, herbs, and spices to make it taste delicious. Once you smell and taste this aromatic blend of spices, fruit, and nuts, you will be transported to a Moroccan souk. I add the garbanzo beans both for protein and texture. This pairs well with Moroccan Chicken (page 112) as well as with grilled chicken, grilled fish, or a roasted cauliflower steak. **MAKES 8 SERVINGS**

¼ cup unsalted butter

2 tablespoons chopped shallots

1 tablespoon Asheville Bee Charmer's Chai-Infused Honey

1 teaspoon kosher salt

½ teaspoon ground ginger

½ teaspoon ground turmeric

½ teaspoon ground cumin

½ teaspoon paprika

½ teaspoon red pepper flakes

2 cups unsalted or low-sodium vegetable stock

½ cup sliced almonds

½ cup currants

1 (15-ounce) can garbanzo beans, drained and rinsed

2 cups quick-cooking couscous

Melt the butter in a medium saucepan set over medium-high heat. Add the shallots and sweat them, stirring occasionally, for about 3 minutes, until they are soft and translucent. Add the honey, salt, ginger, turmeric, cumin, paprika, and red pepper flakes and cook, stirring constantly, for 1 minute, until the onions are fragrant. Add the vegetable stock, almonds, currants, and garbanzo beans. Bring the mixture to a boil, then add the couscous and stir.

Remove the pan from the heat, cover it, and let it stand for 5 to 7 minutes, until all the water has been absorbed. Fluff the couscous with a fork and serve immediately. Store leftover couscous in an airtight container in the refrigerator for 4 to 5 days.

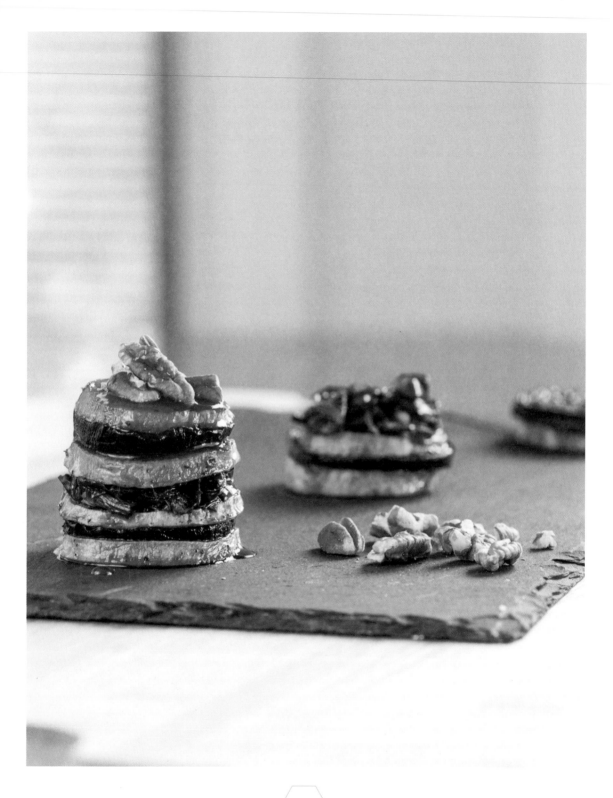

SWEET POTATO NAPOLEON

Beautifully stacked vegetables can make even the simplest preparations look elegant. The colors in this stack are bright and vibrant and the flavor is robust—the naturally sweet beets and potatoes are offset by the bitterness of the chard. Add a drizzle of orange sauce and roasted pecans for additional flavor and crunch and you have a really satisfying side dish. I have substituted sautéed spinach or kale for the chard, and either one works just as well. ✑ **MAKES 6 NAPOLEONS**

¼ cup + 2 tablespoons olive oil, divided

¼ cup carrot honey, divided

1 teaspoon kosher salt, divided

½ teaspoon freshly ground black pepper, divided

2 large sweet potatoes, peeled and cut into 24 (¼-inch-thick) slices

2 red beets, peeled and cut into 12 (¼-inch-thick) slices

1 bunch Swiss chard, stemmed, leaves ripped into small pieces

¾ cup freshly squeezed orange juice

2 tablespoons apple cider vinegar

¼ cup + 2 tablespoons unsalted, toasted pecans, roughly chopped

Preheat the oven to 450°F. Line two baking sheets with parchment paper and set them aside.

To make the marinade, whisk together ¼ cup of the oil, 2 tablespoons of the honey, ½ teaspoon of the salt, and ¼ teaspoon of the pepper in a small bowl. Place the sweet potatoes in a medium bowl. Add the marinade and toss to coat well. Transfer the sweet potatoes to one of the prepared baking sheets. Do not wipe out the bowl.

Place the beets in the same bowl, which should still contain the marinade, and toss to coat completely. Transfer them to the second prepared baking sheet.

Roast the sweet potatoes and beets for 15 minutes, or until the potatoes are golden brown and both vegetables are fork tender. Remove the baking sheets from the oven and set them aside.

In the meantime, heat the remaining 2 tablespoons of oil in a large sauté pan over medium-high heat until it's hot but not yet smoking. Add the Swiss chard leaves, the remaining ½ teaspoon of salt, and the remaining ¼ teaspoon of pepper and sauté for about 5 minutes, or until the chard is cooked through and no longer bitter. Remove the pan from the heat and set it aside.

To make the sauce, heat the orange juice, vinegar, and the remaining 2 tablespoons of honey in a small saucepan set over high heat. Bring the mixture to a boil and let it reduce by half. Remove the pan from the heat and set it aside.

To assemble the napoleons, place one slice of sweet potato on each of six plates. Place one slice of beet on top of each sweet potato slice, and repeat with another slice of sweet potato to cover the beet. Divide the chard evenly among the six stacks. Top the chard in each stack with another slice of sweet potato, another slice of beet, and a final slice of sweet potato. Sprinkle each napoleon with 1 tablespoon of chopped pecans. Drizzle each with 1 tablespoon of orange sauce and serve immediately. Store leftover stacks in an airtight container in the refrigerator for up to 4 days.

GINGER ORANGE MASHED SWEET POTATOES

If you want to make mashed potatoes healthier, use sweet potatoes. They don't quite get the same creaminess of regular mashed potatoes, but they are so flavorful, particularly with the addition of orange and ginger. You can eat these and not feel guilty. ❧ **MAKES 4 SERVINGS**

2 large sweet potatoes, peeled and cut into 1-inch cubes

1 tablespoon unsalted butter

¼ cup freshly squeezed orange juice

1 tablespoon ginger-infused honey

1 teaspoon orange blossom honey

½ teaspoon freshly grated orange zest

½ teaspoon ground ginger

1 teaspoon kosher salt

¼ teaspoon freshly ground black pepper

Place the sweet potatoes in a large saucepan with enough cold water to cover them by 1 inch. Bring the water to a boil over high heat and let the potatoes boil for 10 minutes, or until they are fork tender.

Meanwhile, combine the butter, orange juice, ginger honey, and orange blossom honey in a small saucepan over low heat and cook for 3 to 5 minutes, or until the mixture is heated through.

When the potatoes are done, immediately drain them, transfer them to a large bowl, and mash them with a potato masher. Add the orange juice mixture, orange zest, ginger, salt, and pepper. Stir well and serve immediately. Store leftover sweet potatoes in an airtight container in the refrigerator for up to 5 days.

APPLE AND SAGE BUCKWHEAT

This is great as a gluten-free stuffing alternative for Thanksgiving or Christmas, but you don't need the excuse of a holiday to make it—it's a perfect fall side dish. The buckwheat has a distinct taste, like dark toasted bread or a hoppy IPA. If you prefer, try quinoa, farro, or millet instead. *MAKES 8 SERVINGS*

3 cups water

1½ cups uncooked whole-grain buckwheat groats

1½ teaspoons kosher salt, divided

2 tablespoons olive oil

1 large yellow onion, cut into ¼-inch cubes (about 2 cups)

1 large Braeburn apple, cut into ¼-inch cubes (about 1½ cups)

2 stalks celery, cut into ¼-inch cubes

3 cloves garlic, minced

1 teaspoon dried sage

¼ teaspoon freshly ground black pepper

2 tablespoons sage honey

½ cup salted, roasted pumpkin seeds

Bring the water to a boil in a medium saucepan set over medium high heat. Add the buckwheat and 1 teaspoon of the salt. Bring the water back to a boil, then cover the pan, reduce the heat to low, and simmer for 10 minutes. Remove the pan from the heat, leaving the lid on, and let the buckwheat steam for 15 minutes.

In a large sauté pan, combine the onion, apple, celery, and garlic and sauté for 8 to 10 minutes, until the vegetables and apple are softened and starting to brown slightly. Add the sage, the remaining ½ teaspoon of salt, the pepper, and the honey and cook for 1 to 2 minutes. Remove the pan from the heat.

Transfer the warm buckwheat to a large bowl. Add the onion mixture and pumpkin seeds. Toss and serve. Store leftovers in an airtight container in the refrigerator for up to 5 days.

TUSCAN FARRO

Farro, a type of wheat, is used frequently in Italian and German cuisine but isn't used much in American cuisine. It's a shame, as cooked farro has an interesting chewy, nutty quality. This is a nice summer dish, particularly when you have in-season tomatoes and fresh herbs. I often make this for picnics, as it is at its best served at room temperature. **MAKES 4 TO 6 SERVINGS**

1 cup uncooked farro

3 cups unsalted or low-sodium vegetable stock

¼ cup olive oil

¼ cup freshly squeezed lemon juice

½ tablespoon Tasmanian leatherwood honey

1½ teaspoons kosher salt

½ teaspoon freshly ground black pepper

2 cloves garlic, minced

½ cup green onions, sliced ⅛ inch thick on the bias

½ cup toasted pine nuts

8 ounces grape tomatoes, halved lengthwise

½ cup roughly chopped fresh flat-leaf parsley leaves

½ cup fresh basil leaves, cut into chiffonade

½ cup fresh mint leaves, cut into chiffonade

Rinse the farro and set it aside.

In a small saucepan set over high heat, bring the stock to a boil. Add the farro and stir. Cover the pan, reduce the heat to low, and simmer for 15 minutes. Remove the pan from the heat, leaving the lid on, and let the farro steam for 10 minutes. Drain off any excess liquid and set the farro aside to cool.

To make the dressing, whisk together the olive oil, lemon juice, honey, salt, and pepper in a small bowl and set it aside.

Transfer the cooled farro to a medium bowl. Add the garlic, green onions, pine nuts, tomatoes, parsley, basil, and mint. Add the dressing and mix, making sure everything is well coated. Serve the farro at room temperature. Store leftovers in an airtight container in the refrigerator for up to 2 days.

Pictured on p. 108

JALAPEÑO CHEDDAR CORN BREAD

Earlier this year, Kim and I took a little road trip from Michigan to Asheville. We stopped at her parents' house in Kentucky on the way, and I took out all of her mom's recipes—it's wonderful to explore generations of recipes. Like many family recipes, the measurements were a bit inaccurate, but now I have the best recipe for corn bread. Thanks, Mrs. Allen! ❧ **MAKES 20 SQUARES OF CORN BREAD (8 TO 10 SERVINGS)**

1 cup fine yellow cornmeal

1 teaspoon kosher salt

3 teaspoons baking powder

2 large eggs

1 cup sour cream

2 tablespoons Asheville Bee Charmer's Smokin' Hot Honey (chipotle-infused honey)

½ cup grapeseed oil

1 cup canned cream-style corn

1 (4-ounce) can minced jalapeños

1 cup grated sharp cheddar

Honey Butter (page 177), for serving

Preheat the oven to 350°F. Place a 9 × 13-inch baking pan in the oven to warm.

In a large bowl, mix together the cornmeal, salt, baking powder, eggs, sour cream, honey, oil, and creamed corn until everything is well incorporated.

Remove the pan from the oven and grease it with nonstick cooking spray. Pour half of the batter into the pan. Sprinkle the jalapeños evenly on top, followed by the cheddar. Add the rest of the batter, making sure to fully cover the jalapeños and cheddar.

Bake for 40 to 45 minutes, or until the corn bread is golden brown and a toothpick inserted into the center comes out clean. Remove the corn bread from the oven and let it cool for at least 15 minutes before slicing. Serve slightly warm or at room temperature with the Honey Butter. Store leftover corn bread in an airtight container at room temperature for 1 to 2 days or in the freezer for up to 3 months.

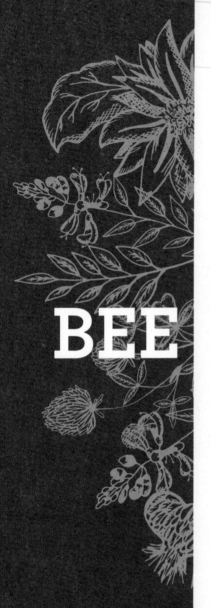

BEE Sweet

CHAPTER 6

Desserts

S'MORES WITH HOMEMADE HONEY GRAHAM CRACKERS

I've never met anyone who doesn't have a great s'mores memory, whether it's from camp, their backyard, or their kitchen. When I was teaching at The Kids' Table, we made graham crackers, and I've never bought graham crackers since. This is a modified version of that recipe. What really makes the recipe special is the meadowfoam honey in the final product. Trust me, your big kids will love these as much as your little kids do! **☙ MAKES 16 S'MORES**

¼ cup unsalted butter, at room temperature

¼ cup firmly packed dark brown sugar

2 tablespoons grapeseed oil

3 tablespoons wildflower honey

1 tablespoon unsweetened applesauce

½ teaspoon pure vanilla extract

½ teaspoon ground ginger

¼ teaspoon baking soda

¼ teaspoon kosher salt

1¼ cups whole wheat flour

2 tablespoons + 2 teaspoons meadowfoam honey

5 tablespoons + 1 teaspoon bittersweet chocolate chips

16 large marshmallows

Preheat the oven to 350°F. Cut 16 (5 × 3-inch) rectangles of parchment paper and set them aside.

In a medium bowl, stir together the butter and brown sugar with a spatula until well incorporated. Add the oil, wildflower honey, applesauce, vanilla, ginger, baking soda, and salt and stir well. Add the flour and stir until just incorporated.

Divide the dough into 16 equal pieces. Take one piece and place it on one of the prepared parchment rectangles. Using the parchment paper as a guide, shape the dough into a rectangle by rolling it out until it's about ¼ inch thick and 4 × 2 inches in size. With a butter knife, score the dough about three-fourths of the way through so that each cracker is a 2-inch square. Poke a few holes in each cracker with a fork. Repeat with the remaining 15 dough balls.

Transfer the crackers with their parchment paper to a baking sheet. Bake for 7 to 8 minutes, or until the edges are lightly browned. Remove the crackers from the oven and transfer them to a wire rack to cool.

Turn on the broiler. Line a baking sheet with aluminum foil and set it aside.

To assemble the s'mores, break each cooled cracker into 2-inch squares. Spread ½ teaspoon of the meadowfoam honey on 16 of the squares. Place 1 teaspoon of the bittersweet chocolate chips on each honey-smeared cracker. Place 1 marshmallow on each mound of chocolate chips. Transfer the 16 crackers to the prepared baking sheet.

Broil for 30 to 60 seconds, or until the marshmallows are lightly browned. Remove the baking sheet from the oven and top each s'more with one of the remaining crackers. Serve immediately. Store any leftover graham crackers in an airtight container at room temperature for 2 to 3 days.

MEXICAN CHOCOLATE COOKIES

Mexican hot chocolate combines the flavors of rich, dark chocolate, spicy chile, cinnamon, and vanilla. Why not use them in a cookie? These cake-like cookies are so rich, even fellow chocoholics find it difficult to eat more than one at a time! They freeze well, too.
MAKES ABOUT 40 COOKIES

15 ounces bittersweet chocolate chips (at least 67% cacao), divided

1 stick (½ cup) unsalted butter, cut into ½-inch pieces

3 large eggs

¼ cup Asheville Bee Charmer's Cocoa-Infused Honey

¼ cup Asheville Bee Charmer's Firecracker Hot Honey

¼ cup firmly packed light brown sugar

2½ teaspoons finely ground dark-roast coffee beans

1 teaspoon pure vanilla extract

1 cup all-purpose flour

¼ cup unsweetened cocoa powder

½ teaspoon baking powder

½ teaspoon kosher salt

½ teaspoon ancho chili powder

½ teaspoon ground cinnamon

Preheat the oven to 350°F. Line two baking sheets with parchment paper and set them aside.

In a metal bowl over simmering water or in a double boiler, melt 9 ounces of the chocolate chips with the butter, stirring until smooth. Remove from the heat and set aside.

In the bowl of a stand mixer fitted with the whisk attachment, beat the eggs, honeys, brown sugar, and ground coffee for 3 to 5 minutes, until well mixed and lightened in color. Add the melted chocolate mixture and the vanilla and beat until thoroughly combined.

In a medium bowl, whisk together the flour, cocoa powder, baking powder, salt, chili powder, and cinnamon. Add this mixture to the chocolate mixture and stir until just combined. Remove the bowl from the mixer and, with a rubber spatula, fold in the remaining 6 ounces of chocolate chips. Let the batter rest for about 5 minutes.

Using a small portion scoop or a tablespoon measure, portion the cookie dough onto the prepared baking sheets, spacing the cookies about 2 inches apart. Transfer the baking sheets to the oven and bake for 12 to 14 minutes, rotating the sheets halfway through, until the cookies are puffed and cracked on top.

Remove the cookies from the oven and let them cool on the baking sheets for 2 minutes, then transfer them to wire racks to cool completely. Store them in an airtight container at room temperature for up to 5 days or in the freezer for up to 6 months.

Pictured on p. 155

ROSEMARY POLENTA CAKE

I tried polenta cake for the first time a few years ago. The flavor and the texture of the cake are interesting, if a little dense. To lighten things up, I add almond meal, but the flavor of the cornmeal still comes through. With the rich butter taste and the fresh rosemary, you have a cake that's just as good for an afternoon snack as it is for dessert. **MAKES 8 SERVINGS**

¾ cup + 2 tablespoons almond meal

¾ cup + 2 tablespoons fine yellow cornmeal

¾ teaspoon kosher salt

2 sticks (1 cup) unsalted butter, at room temperature

¾ cup + 2 tablespoons raw cane sugar

3 tablespoons Asheville Bee Charmer's Rosemary-Infused Honey

1 tablespoon minced fresh rosemary

1 teaspoon freshly grated orange zest

5 large eggs, at room temperature

Preheat the oven to 325°F. Grease a Bundt pan with nonstick cooking spray and set it aside.

In a small bowl, stir together the almond meal, cornmeal, and salt; set it aside.

In the bowl of a stand mixer fitted with the paddle attachment, combine the butter, sugar, honey, rosemary, and orange zest. Mix on low speed until everything is incorporated. Increase the speed to medium and cream the mixture for 5 minutes, scraping down the sides of the bowl and the paddle at least twice, until the mixture is pale and fluffy.

Reduce the speed to low. Add the eggs, one at a time, making sure each one is fully incorporated before adding the next. Scrape down the sides of the bowl, if necessary. Add the almond meal and cornmeal mixture and mix until just combined.

Pour the batter into the prepared Bundt pan. Bake for about 1 hour, or until the cake is golden brown and a toothpick inserted into the center comes out clean. Remove the cake from the oven and let it cool in the pan for at least 10 minutes, then invert it onto a wire rack to cool completely.

Slice the cake and serve it at room temperature. Store it in an airtight container at room temperature for up to 4 days.

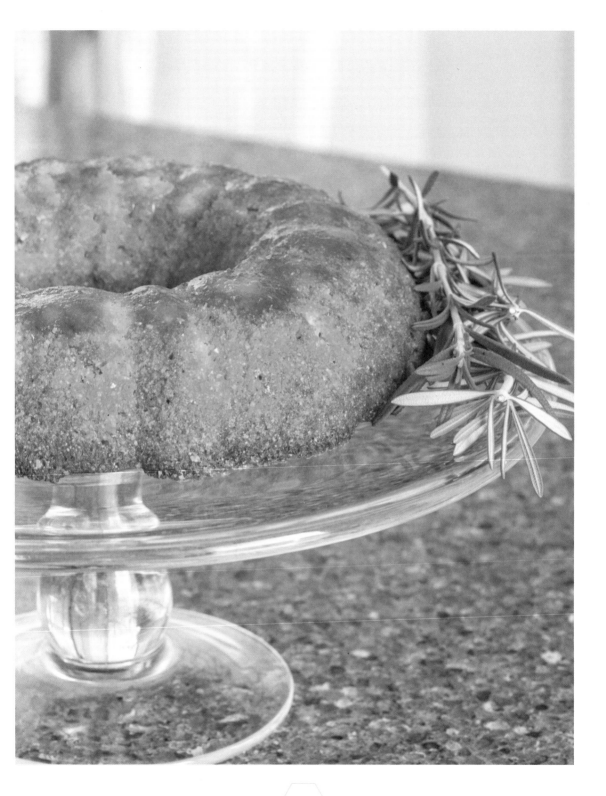

CHOCOLATE AVOCADO MOUSSE

Not only are avocados filled with nutrients and healthy fats, but their creamy, buttery texture also makes them a fat replacer in a lot of recipes. Of course they taste great in guacamole, on salads, and on toast, but they taste even more delicious when mixed with chocolate and honey. This mousse is quick and easy, and it's probably one of the healthiest chocolate desserts you'll ever eat. 🐝 **MAKES ABOUT 2 CUPS**

2 ripe avocados, peeled and pitted

⅓ cup dates, pitted and chopped into ¼-inch cubes

½ cup unsweetened cocoa powder

½ cup Asheville Bee Charmer's Cocoa-Infused Honey

⅓ cup water, divided

Place the avocados, dates, cocoa powder, honey, and 2 tablespoons of the water in a blender. Blend on high, making sure the avocados and dates are fully incorporated. Slowly add the rest of the water, as needed, until the mousse is fully emulsified. It should take about 5 minutes of blending time to get a light and fluffy mousse.

Transfer the mousse to an airtight container and refrigerate until you're ready to serve. It can be stored in an airtight container in the refrigerator for 4 to 5 days.

GRILLED INDIAN FRUIT SALAD WITH SPICED YOGURT

Grilling fruit intensifies its flavor by caramelizing the natural sugars. Adding chai honey to the oil in which you mix the fruit adds a burst of spicy flavor. For a dipping sauce, try mixing some chai honey and Greek yogurt together. You'll love the flavor of the yogurt so much, I bet you'll start eating it even without the fruit! ✺ **MAKES 8 SERVINGS**

FRUIT SALAD

1 (3-pound) pineapple

3 ripe mangoes

3 oranges

¼ cup grapeseed oil

¼ cup Asheville Bee Charmer's Chai-Infused Honey

SPICED YOGURT

2 cups plain Greek yogurt

½ cup Asheville Bee Charmer's Chai-Infused Honey

1 tablespoon + 1 teaspoon freshly grated lime zest, for garnish

Preheat a grill to medium heat. Soak 8 to 10 (8-inch) wooden skewers in water for 10 to 15 minutes.

To make the fruit salad, peel, quarter, and core the pineapple. Cut each quarter in half lengthwise and then cut each piece into 1-inch chunks. Place the pineapple in a large bowl. Peel the mangoes. Cut the flesh off the seeds and chop it into 1-inch chunks. Add the mangoes to the bowl with the pineapple. Peel the oranges. Quarter the oranges lengthwise and cut them into 1-inch chunks. Add the oranges to the bowl with the pineapple and mangoes.

In a small bowl, whisk together the oil and honey. Add this mixture to the fruit and toss to coat completely. Thread the fruit onto skewers. Grill the fruit for 8 to 10 minutes, turning once or twice, until it is nicely browned.

To make the spiced yogurt, whisk together the Greek yogurt and honey.

To serve, divide the yogurt among eight bowls. Top with the grilled fruit and garnish each serving with some lime zest. Serve immediately. Store leftover grilled fruit in an airtight container in the refrigerator for 2 to 3 days.

NOTE *Other fruits that work well with this are bananas, peaches, and nectarines. If you don't have a grill, you can place the fruit on an aluminum foil–lined baking sheet and broil the fruit for 8 to 10 minutes, stirring after 4 to 5 minutes.*

LEMON CURD MERINGUES WITH FRESH BLUEBERRIES

When I lived in England, I became a big fan of lemon curd, and meringue cups are an edible way to serve it with fresh fruit. The sourwood honey in this curd adds great flavor, but it doesn't make it overly sweet. I use Berry Coulis made with blueberries as well as fresh berries to finish off this dessert, which works with both casual and elegant dinners. **MAKES 20 TO 25 MERINGUES**

MERINGUES

4 large egg whites, at room temperature

½ teaspoon cream of tartar

⅛ teaspoon kosher salt

1 cup granulated raw cane sugar

LEMON CURD

2 large eggs

2 large egg yolks

¼ cup sourwood honey

¼ cup + 2 tablespoons freshly squeezed lemon juice

¼ cup raw cane sugar

2 tablespoons freshly grated lemon zest

1 stick (½ cup) cold unsalted butter, cut into small pieces

ASSEMBLY

1 pint blueberries

1½ cups Berry Coulis (page 176), made with blueberries

Preheat the oven to 200°F. Line two baking sheets with parchment paper and set them aside.

To make the meringues, place the egg whites, cream of tartar, and salt in the bowl of a stand mixer fitted with the whisk attachment. Begin beating on low, and gradually increase the speed to high as the whites begin to foam. Gradually add the sugar and continue beating on high speed until the meringue is stiff and glossy.

Transfer the meringue to a piping bag fitted with a large star tip. Pipe a 2-inch circle onto one of the prepared baking sheets and fill it completely with meringue, then pipe the meringue two or three times around the edge of the circle, depending on how high you want the shell to be. Repeat with the remaining meringue, making 19 to 24 more shells.

Transfer the meringue shells to the oven and bake for 1½ hours. Turn the oven off and let the meringue shells sit for at least 1 hour. It's important that you don't open the oven. The meringues should still be bright white and the outside should feel crisp to the touch. Remove the meringue shells from the oven and let them cool completely.

While the meringues are baking, make the lemon curd. Whisk together the eggs, egg yolks, honey, lemon juice, sugar, and lemon zest in a small heatproof bowl.

In a medium saucepan set over medium heat, bring about an inch of water to a simmer. Set the heatproof bowl on top of the saucepan, making sure the water doesn't touch the bottom of the bowl.

Whisk the egg mixture constantly until the curd thickens and an instant-read thermometer inserted into the curd registers 180°F. Remove the bowl from the heat and whisk in the butter. Transfer the curd to a cool bowl and chill it quickly in ice water, stirring every few minutes. Once it has cooled, refrigerate the curd.

To assemble the dessert, spoon 1 tablespoon of the Berry Coulis on each individual plate. Place a meringue cup on top and fill it with lemon curd. Top with some fresh blueberries and serve immediately.

 NOTE *The meringue cups can be prepared up to a week in advance. Just store them in an airtight container at room temperature. The lemon curd can also be made up to a week in advance and stored in an airtight container in the refrigerator.*

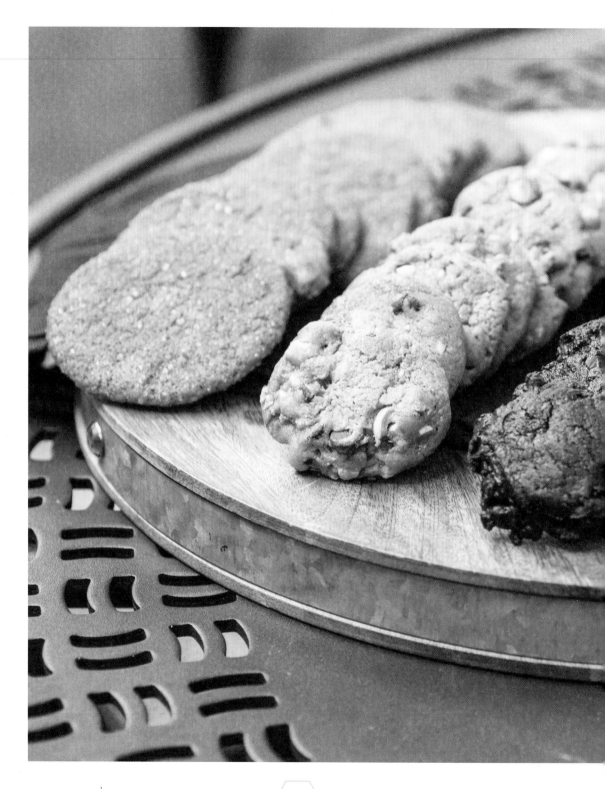

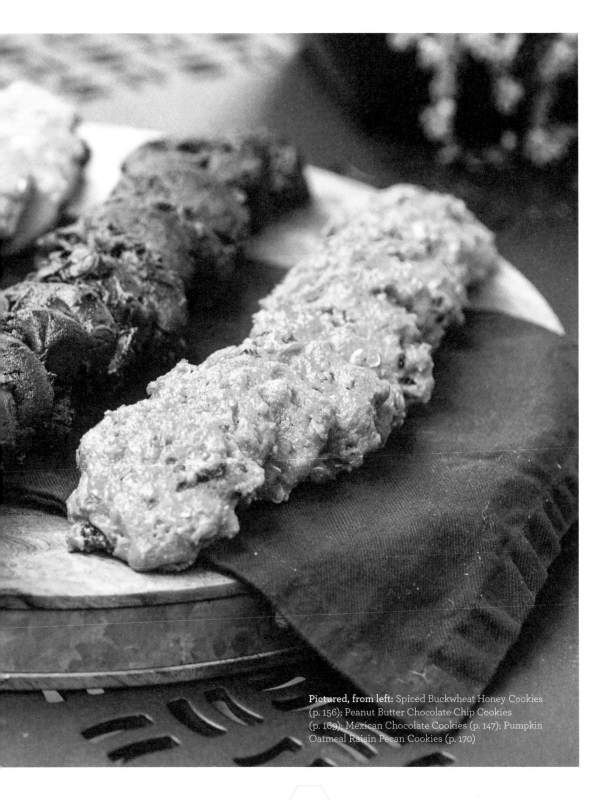

Pictured, from left: Spiced Buckwheat Honey Cookies (p. 156); Peanut Butter Chocolate Chip Cookies (p. 169); Mexican Chocolate Cookies (p. 147); Pumpkin Oatmeal Raisin Pecan Cookies (p. 170)

SPICED BUCKWHEAT HONEY COOKIES

These are inspired by molasses cookies, which can be a bit cloying at times. Using the buckwheat honey gives them a much mellower flavor. Don't let the smell of the buckwheat honey turn you off while you're making these cookies. As they bake, the smell goes away and you're left with a moist, spicy, and sweet cookie. ❧ **MAKES 40 COOKIES**

1½ sticks (¾ cup) unsalted butter, at room temperature

1 cup firmly packed light brown sugar

¼ cup buckwheat honey

1 large egg

2½ teaspoons baking soda

½ teaspoon ground cloves

½ teaspoon ground nutmeg

1 teaspoon ground ginger

¼ teaspoon ground cardamom

½ teaspoon ground allspice

½ teaspoon kosher salt

1 cup all-purpose flour

1 cup whole wheat flour

½ cup raw cane sugar

Preheat the oven to 350°F. Line two baking sheets with parchment paper and set them aside.

In a large bowl, mix the butter, brown sugar, and honey with a wooden spoon until well blended. Add the egg and blend well. Add the baking soda, cloves, nutmeg, ginger, cardamom, allspice, and salt and mix well. Add the all-purpose and whole wheat flours and stir until just combined.

Place the raw cane sugar in a small bowl.

Using a small cookie scoop, form 40 balls of dough. If you don't have a cookie scoop, use a tablespoon measure and roll each scoop into a ball with your hands. Roll each dough ball in the cane sugar. Place the balls on the prepared baking sheets, spacing them 2 inches apart (the cookies will spread).

Transfer the baking sheets to the oven and bake the cookies for 9 to 11 minutes, or until they slightly crack on top. I like to rotate the baking sheets after 5 minutes. Remove the cookies from the oven and let them cool on the baking sheets for 5 minutes, then transfer them to wire racks to cool completely. Store the cookies in an airtight container at room temperature for up to 4 days or in the freezer for up to 6 months.

Pictured on p. 154

CHOCOLATE HAZELNUT PINWHEELS

These pinwheels showcase the delectable flavor combination of chocolate and hazelnut. And since they contain bittersweet chocolate, they don't get overly sweet. These are just as good with a cup of coffee in the morning as they are with a glass of red wine after dinner. ❧ **MAKES 56 PINWHEELS**

¼ cup unsalted butter

¼ cup Asheville Bee Charmer's Cocoa-Infused Honey

All-purpose flour, for dusting

1 pound puff pastry, thawed and cut in half

1½ cups unsalted, roasted hazelnuts, roughly chopped

1½ cups bittersweet chocolate chips

Heat the butter and honey in a small saucepan over medium heat for about 5 minutes, stirring occasionally, until the butter is melted and the honey is completely incorporated.

Dust a clean work surface with the all-purpose flour. With a rolling pin, roll out one piece of puff pastry into a 9 × 15-inch rectangle. Using a pastry brush, brush half of the honey-butter mixture on the piece of puff pastry, making sure to fully cover it. Sprinkle on ¾ cup of the hazelnuts and ¾ cup of the chocolate chips, leaving a 1-inch strip along one 15-inch side. Begin rolling the puff pastry from the other 15-inch side, making sure to roll the dough fairly tightly. Wrap the rolled dough with plastic wrap. Repeat the process with the other piece of puff pastry and the remaining honey-butter mixture, hazelnuts, and chocolate chips. Refrigerate the rolled dough for at least 2 hours, or until firm.

Preheat the oven to 400°F. Line two baking sheets with parchment paper and set them aside.

Unwrap one of the chocolate hazelnut rolls. With a sharp knife, cut ½ inch off of each end and discard. Cut the roll into 28 (½-inch-thick) slices. Repeat this process with the second roll. Place the pinwheel slices on the prepared baking sheets, spacing them about 1½ inches apart.

Transfer the pinwheels to the oven and bake for 8 minutes, then rotate the baking sheets and bake for another 8 to 9 minutes, or until the cookies are golden brown. Remove the baking sheets from the oven and transfer the cookies to wire racks to cool. Serve immediately or store the cookies in an airtight container at room temperature for up to 7 days.

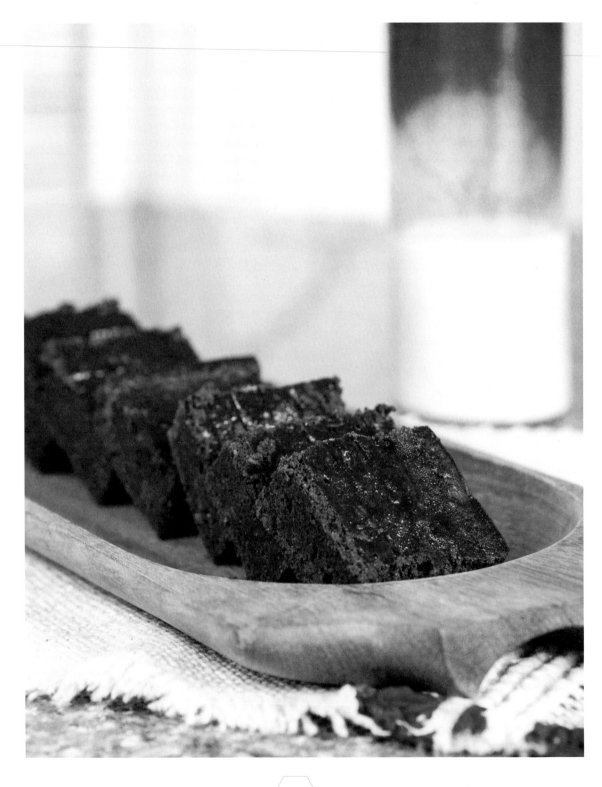

BLACK BEAN BROWNIES

The first time I taught a version of this recipe at The Kids' Table, I was very skeptical that the kids would even try these brownies. However, I misjudged the power of chocolate. Not only did they try them, they liked them. These taste like regular, dense brownies, but they are so much healthier due to the black beans and applesauce. Make them for your friends and family; just don't tell anyone what's in them until they've had a taste! *MAKES 24 BROWNIES*

1 cup bittersweet chocolate chips, divided

1 (15-ounce) can black beans, drained and rinsed

½ cup unsweetened applesauce

½ cup olive oil

4 large eggs

⅔ cup firmly packed dark brown sugar

½ cup Asheville Bee Charmer's Cocoa-Infused Honey

½ cup unsweetened cocoa powder

2 teaspoons pure vanilla extract

⅔ cup all-purpose flour

1 teaspoon baking powder

¼ teaspoon kosher salt

Preheat the oven to 350°F. Grease a 9 × 13-inch pan with nonstick cooking spray and set it aside.

In a double boiler or in a microwave, melt ½ cup of the chocolate chips; set it aside.

In a blender, combine the black beans, applesauce, and olive oil. Blend until smooth, about 2 minutes. Add the eggs, brown sugar, honey, cocoa powder, and vanilla. Blend until smooth, another 1 to 2 minutes. Add the melted chocolate and blend until it is fully incorporated, about 1 minute longer.

In a medium bowl, whisk together the flour, baking powder, and salt. Add the chocolate mixture to the flour mixture. Make sure to use a rubber spatula to get all of the chocolate mixture out of the blender! Stir until the flour just disappears. Fold in the remaining ½ cup of chocolate chips.

Pour the batter into the prepared pan. Transfer the pan to the oven and bake for 30 minutes, or until a toothpick inserted into the center of the brownie comes out clean.

Remove the brownie from the oven and let it cool in the pan for 10 minutes, then invert it onto a wire rack to cool completely. Cut the brownie into 24 pieces and serve. Store leftover brownies in an airtight container at room temperature for 3 to 4 days or in the freezer for up to 6 months.

CHOCOLATE PISTACHIO BAKLAVA

I find a lot of baklava to be overly sweet, so I've added bittersweet chocolate to this version. Pistachios taste wonderful with the chocolate, but you could use walnuts, too. Baklava is one of those desserts that anyone can make, and it's fun to make with the kids! ❧ **MAKES 32 SQUARES**

FILLING

3 cups salted, roasted pistachios, shelled and finely chopped

1 cup bittersweet chocolate chips, melted

¼ cup unseasoned breadcrumbs

3 tablespoons acacia honey

1 teaspoon ground cinnamon

2 sticks (1 cup) unsalted butter, melted

ASSEMBLY

2 sticks (1 cup) unsalted butter, melted

10–12 ounces (14 × 18-inch sheets) phyllo dough, thawed in the refrigerator (see Note on page 48)

SYRUP

2 cups water

1 cup acacia honey

2 whole cloves

1 cinnamon stick

1 tablespoon freshly squeezed lemon juice

Preheat the oven to 350°F. Grease a 9 × 14-inch baking dish with butter and set it aside.

To make the filling, mix together the pistachios, melted chocolate, breadcrumbs, honey, cinnamon, and melted butter in a medium bowl. Set it aside.

To assemble the baklava, lay one sheet of phyllo on the bottom of the prepared baking dish. Brush it lightly with the melted butter. Repeat four more times, so that you have five sheets of phyllo on the bottom of the dish. Spread one-fourth of the filling all over the dough. Lay a sheet of phyllo on top of the filling and brush it with the melted butter. Repeat this process four more times so you have a total of five phyllo sheets on top of the filling. Repeat the layering process until you've used all of the filling.

Place one sheet of phyllo on the final layer of filling and brush it with the melted butter. Repeat five more times so that you have a total of six phyllo sheets on top. Brush the top very generously with the melted butter.

Transfer the baklava to the oven and bake for 50 to 60 minutes, or until it is golden brown.

While the baklava is baking, make the syrup. Heat the water and honey in a medium saucepan over medium-high heat, stirring frequently, until the honey has dissolved. Add the cloves and cinnamon stick. Bring the mixture to a boil, reduce the heat to low, and let it simmer for 10 minutes. Remove and discard the cloves and cinnamon stick. Stir in the lemon juice.

Remove the baklava from the oven and place it on a wire rack to cool. Pour the syrup over the entire dish of baklava. The syrup will be absorbed as the baklava cools. Once it's at room temperature, cut the baklava into 32 squares and serve. Store leftovers in the baking dish, covered tightly with plastic wrap, for 4 to 5 days.

ROASTED PINEAPPLE CHAI SORBET

One time when I was making Grilled Indian Fruit Salad (page 151), I snuck some of the pineapple and thought, "Wouldn't that make a great frozen treat?" I decided to turn the pineapple into an easy-to-make sorbet without using an ice cream maker. It's refreshing and can satisfy a sweet craving in a flash—plus, there's no added sugar! ❧ **MAKES ABOUT 2 CUPS**

2 tablespoons Asheville Bee Charmer's Chai-Infused Honey, divided

1 tablespoon grapeseed oil

1 small pineapple, peeled, quartered, cored, and cut into ½-inch-thick slices

1 teaspoon freshly squeezed lemon juice

½ cup water

Preheat the oven to 450°F. Line a baking sheet with parchment paper and set it aside.

In a small bowl, whisk together 1 tablespoon plus 1 teaspoon of the honey and the grapeseed oil. Place the pineapple slices on the prepared baking sheet. Brush both sides with the honey-oil mixture. Transfer the pineapple to the oven and roast for 25 minutes, or until golden brown. Remove the pineapple from the oven and let it cool.

In a blender, combine the cooled pineapple with the remaining 2 teaspoons of honey, the lemon juice, and the water. Blend on high until the purée is very smooth. Pour the purée in a thin layer on a nonstick baking sheet. Freeze for 45 minutes, or until solid.

Break the frozen sorbet into small chunks and transfer it to the blender. Blend on high until the mixture is whipped, about 2 minutes. Serve immediately or refreeze the sorbet in an airtight container for up to 3 months.

the asheville bee charmer cookbook

BERRY CHIA SEED PUDDING

When I was in culinary school, I did a project with two classmates on chia seeds, one of the most nutritious foods in existence. What's really interesting about them is how they absorb liquid and become almost gelatinous. I like eating this pudding for a light dessert, but it also makes a delicious and nutritious breakfast. ❧ **MAKES 4 SERVINGS**

1 cup unsweetened coconut milk	**½ teaspoon pure vanilla extract**
1 cup unsweetened almond milk	**¼ cup blueberry honey**
½ cup chia seeds	**2 cups fresh or frozen blueberries**

In a medium bowl, whisk together the coconut milk, almond milk, chia seeds, vanilla, and honey. Let the mixture sit for 10 minutes, then whisk it again to break up any lumps. Stir in the berries. Cover and refrigerate the mixture for at least 3 hours or ideally overnight. Stir well before serving. Store leftover pudding in an airtight container in the refrigerator for up to 4 days.

NOTE *If you don't like blueberries, you can use blackberries or raspberries and the corresponding honey varietal. You can also add chopped nuts, if you like. Other fruits that are great to use for this pudding are banana, mango, and/or pineapple.*

BLACKBERRY MEAD POACHED PEARS WITH HONEY RICOTTA

One time when I went to visit the Queen Bees in Asheville, we went to Bee & Bramble to taste mead, including a blackberry variety. That was the genesis of this recipe. I usually use a nice red wine to poach pears, but the mead, mixed with some fresh berries, added a unique flavor and gorgeous color. Served with some ricotta and a drizzle of blackberry honey, this is a flavorful, eye-catching dessert. **MAKES 4 SERVINGS**

2 cups blackberry mead

¾ cup blackberry honey, divided

Peel of 1 lemon

Heaping ½ cup fresh or frozen blackberries, smashed

2 cups water

4 ripe but firm Bosc or Anjou pears, peeled and cored

2 cups whole-milk ricotta

In a medium saucepan, combine the mead, ½ cup of the honey, the lemon peel, the blackberries, and the water. Carefully stand the pears upright in the liquid and bring the liquid to a boil over medium heat. Reduce the heat to low and simmer for 15 minutes, or until a paring knife can be easily inserted into the pears.

Remove the pan from the heat and let the pears cool in the cooking liquid. Cover and refrigerate the pears until they are completely chilled. Remove the pears from the cooking liquid; discard the cooking liquid. Before serving, let the pears come back to room temperature.

To serve the pears, place ½ cup of the ricotta in each of four small bowls. Drizzle each bowl with 1 tablespoon of the remaining blackberry honey, top with a pear, and serve. Store leftover cooked pears separately in an airtight container for 2 to 3 days.

NOTE *Mead is often sold at farmers' markets, although you can usually find it at liquor stores, too. If you can't find blackberry mead, try this recipe with a different kind.*

CHAI PUMPKIN PIE

Growing up, my mom made a wonderful pumpkin chiffon pie for Thanksgiving every year. What made it special was that it had a light, airy quality, despite the density of the pumpkin. This pie isn't quite as light as my mom's, but the addition of coconut milk yogurt cuts through the heaviness of the pumpkin purée. The chai spice and the pecan oat crust add unique twists to an American classic. **MAKES 8 SERVINGS**

CRUST

2 cups pecan halves

1 cup gluten-free rolled oats (not quick cooking)

¼ cup unsalted butter, cut into ½-inch pieces

5 pitted dates

1 tablespoon Asheville Bee Charmer's Chai-Infused Honey

2 tablespoons firmly packed dark brown sugar

1 teaspoon kosher salt

FILLING

15 ounces fresh or canned pumpkin purée

¾ cup firmly packed dark brown sugar

1 teaspoon ground ginger

½ teaspoon kosher salt

1¼ cups unsweetened coconut milk yogurt

2 tablespoons Asheville Bee Charmer's Chai-Infused Honey

2 large eggs

Preheat the oven to 350°F.

To make the crust, place all the ingredients in the bowl of a food processor. Mix until everything is finely chopped and fully incorporated. Press the dough into a deep-dish pie pan. Make sure to firmly press it down. I use a ¼-cup measuring cup to press the bottom first, from the center moving out, and then the sides.

To make the filling, whisk together the pumpkin purée, brown sugar, ground ginger, salt, yogurt, honey, and eggs in a large bowl. Pour the filling into the prepared crust.

Bake for 50 minutes, or until the center jiggles only slightly when you move the pan. The filling will firm up as it cools. Check the pie at 30 minutes and 40 minutes. If the crust looks like it is starting to brown too much, cover the pie loosely with aluminum foil.

Remove the pie from the oven and let it cool on a wire rack. Serve at room temperature. Store the pie, covered with plastic wrap, in the refrigerator for 4 to 5 days.

CANDIED ORANGE OLIVE OIL ALMOND CAKE

For years, I've been making a flourless orange cake for Passover. Every year I think to myself, "I should make it more often." Then I saw a *Bon Appétit* recipe for olive oil cake with candied oranges on top. This cake combines both recipes—and it happens to be dairy free. When you are craving something sweet, but want something light, this is the cake for you. ❧ **MAKES 8 TO 10 SERVINGS**

SYRUP

½ cup raw cane sugar

½ cup orange blossom honey

2 cups water

1 navel orange, cut into ⅛-inch-thick slices

CAKE

2 cups almond flour

1½ teaspoons baking powder

1 teaspoon ground cardamom

½ teaspoon kosher salt

¼ teaspoon baking soda

¼ cup raw cane sugar

½ cup olive oil

3 large eggs

½ cup unsweetened coconut milk yogurt

1½ tablespoons freshly grated orange zest

1 teaspoon pure vanilla extract

To make the syrup, combine the sugar, honey, and water in a small saucepan set over medium-high heat. Bring the mixture to a boil, stirring until the sugar dissolves. Add the orange slices, reduce the heat to medium low, and simmer until the syrup is reduced by half, about 45 minutes.

Transfer the orange slices to a parchment paper–lined baking sheet. Continue simmering the syrup until it is reduced by half again, about 30 minutes (you should have about ¾ cup left). Remove the syrup from the heat and set it aside.

Preheat the oven to 350°F. Grease a 10-inch springform pan with nonstick cooking spray.

To make the batter, place the flour, baking powder, cardamom, salt, baking soda, and sugar in a large bowl. Stir to mix well. Add the olive oil, eggs, yogurt, orange zest, and vanilla. Mix well, making sure everything is thoroughly incorporated.

Pour the batter into the prepared pan and place it on a baking sheet. Bake for 35 minutes, or until the cake is golden brown and a toothpick inserted into the center comes out clean.

Remove the cake from the oven. Poke small holes in the cake with a toothpick. (Really make a lot of holes.) Pour ¼ cup of the syrup over the cake. Transfer the cake in its pan to a wire rack to cool.

After the cake has cooled, run a butter knife around the edge of the pan and open the springform pan. Place all the candied orange slices on top of the cake. Slice and serve with the remaining syrup. Store the cake in an airtight container in the refrigerator for 4 to 5 days.

MINI CRANBERRY APPLE GALETTES

A couple of years ago, I began focusing on single-serve desserts. These galettes originated as hand pies, which I felt had too much crust and not enough filling, so I turned them into open pies, or galettes. The natural sweetness of the fruit filling is enhanced by a touch of honey. These taste great plain or served with some ice cream or whipped cream. For variation, substitute raisins for the cranberries for an apple strudel galette. ❧ **MAKES 12 SMALL GALETTES**

DOUGH

3 cups all-purpose flour

1 teaspoon raw cane sugar

½ teaspoon kosher salt

2 sticks (1 cup) cold unsalted butter, cut into ½-inch pieces

¼ cup vodka

¼ cup ice water

FILLING

½ pound fresh or frozen cranberries, or 8 ounces dried cranberries

1 pound Braeburn apples, peeled, cored, and cut into ½-inch cubes

1½ teaspoons freshly squeezed lemon juice

2 tablespoons unsalted butter, melted

⅓ cup almond meal

2 tablespoons cranberry honey

½ teaspoon ground ginger

ASSEMBLY

¼ cup unsalted butter, melted

¼ cup raw cane sugar

To make the dough, place the flour, sugar, salt, and butter in a food processor and pulse until the butter is the size of small peas. With the machine running, add the vodka and ice water and blend until the dough comes together.

Divide the dough into two pieces and flatten each into a round disc. Wrap the dough discs in plastic wrap and refrigerate for at least 1 hour.

To make the filling, mix together the cranberries, apples, lemon juice, melted butter, almond meal, honey, and ginger in a large bowl; set it aside.

Preheat the oven to 375°F. Line two baking sheets with parchment paper and set them aside.

To assemble the galettes, on a lightly floured surface, roll out one disc of dough to a ¼-inch thickness. Using a 4-inch round cutter or a small plate, cut out six circles of dough. Fill each circle with ⅓ cup of the filling. Gently lift up the sides of the dough so it partially covers the filling. Repeat with the remaining dough disc and filling and place the formed galettes on the prepared baking sheets.

Brush each galette with 1 teaspoon of the melted butter and sprinkle with 1 teaspoon of the cane sugar.

Transfer the baking sheets to the oven and bake for 35 to 40 minutes, or until the galettes are golden brown. Remove the galettes from the oven and let them cool on the baking sheets for 10 minutes, then transfer them to wire racks to cool completely. Serve at room temperature. Store leftover galettes in an airtight container at room temperature for up to 3 days.

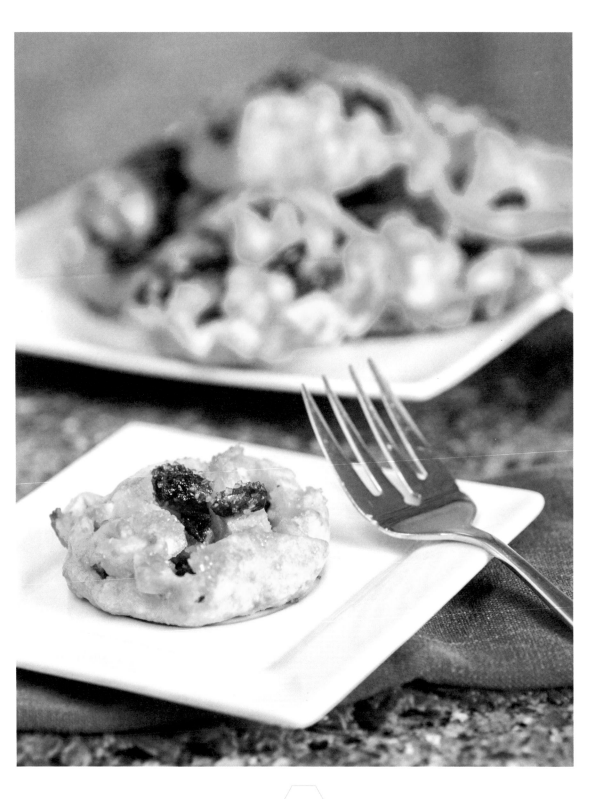

the asheville bee charmer cookbook

APPLE CINNAMON WALNUT CAKE WITH CHAI HONEY GLAZE

I think everyone's mom has a great apple cake recipe. It's usually just apples in a relatively plain cake base. If you want to make it a little more interesting, add honey, nuts, and cinnamon. The chai honey glaze makes this cake extra special. 🐝 **MAKES 8 TO 10 SERVINGS**

CAKE

1 cup raw cane sugar

¼ cup Asheville Bee Charmer's Chai-Infused Honey

½ cup wildflower honey

½ cup grapeseed oil

3 large eggs

2 teaspoons pure vanilla extract

2 teaspoons ground cinnamon

1 teaspoon kosher salt

1 teaspoon baking powder

1 cup almond meal

2 cups all-purpose flour

1 cup chopped walnuts

2 Pink Lady apples, peeled, cored, and cut into ¼-inch cubes (3 cups)

GLAZE

1 cup powdered sugar

2 tablespoons Asheville Bee Charmer's Chai-Infused Honey

2 tablespoons 2% milk

Preheat the oven to 325°F. Grease a Bundt pan with nonstick cooking spray and set it aside.

To make the batter, whisk together the sugar, Chai-Infused Honey, wildflower honey, oil, eggs, and vanilla in a large bowl. Add the cinnamon, salt, baking powder, almond meal, and flour. Stir with a rubber spatula until the dry ingredients are just incorporated. Fold in the walnuts and apples until well mixed.

Transfer the batter to the prepared pan and bake for 1½ hours, or until the cake is well browned and just starting to pull away from the edges, and a toothpick inserted into the center comes out clean.

Remove the cake from the oven and let it cool in its pan for 1 hour, then invert it onto a wire rack and let it cool completely. Once the cake is cool, transfer it to a cake stand or large plate.

To make the glaze, whisk together the sugar, honey, and milk in a small bowl. Pour the glaze over the top of the cake. Slice and serve. Store the cake in an airtight container in the refrigerator for 4 to 5 days.

PEANUT BUTTER CHOCOLATE CHIP COOKIES

Peanut butter and chocolate is a no-brainer flavor combination for desserts, including cookies. When you add honey to the mix, it tastes as if honey-roasted peanuts have been ground into a delicious cookie. They don't spread a lot when you bake them, yet despite this, you end up with a relatively crunchy cookie. These cookies freeze really well. **✿ MAKES 36 TO 38 COOKIES**

½ cup chunky peanut butter, at room temperature

2 tablespoons unsalted butter, at room temperature

½ cup wildflower honey

½ cup firmly packed dark brown sugar

1 large egg

1 teaspoon pure vanilla extract

1 cup all-purpose flour

½ cup whole wheat flour

¾ teaspoon baking soda

1 teaspoon kosher salt

1 cup semi-sweet chocolate chips

½ cup unsalted, roasted peanuts, chopped

In the bowl of a stand mixer fitted with a paddle attachment, combine the peanut butter, butter, honey, and brown sugar. Cream the mixture on medium speed for 10 minutes, or until fluffy and almost doubled in volume. Reduce the speed to low, add the egg and vanilla, and mix until they are incorporated. Carefully add the all-purpose flour, whole wheat flour, baking soda, and salt and mix until just combined. Add the chocolate chips and peanuts and mix until well incorporated.

Remove the bowl from the mixer, cover it with plastic wrap, and chill the batter for 1 hour in the refrigerator.

Preheat the oven to 350°F. Line two baking sheets with parchment paper.

Roll 1 tablespoon of the dough into a small ball. Place it on a prepared baking sheet and flatten it slightly. Repeat this process with the rest of the dough, making sure to space the cookies 2 inches apart on the baking sheets.

Transfer the cookies to the oven, bake for 5 minutes, and then rotate the baking sheets. Bake for another 5 minutes, or until the cookies are golden brown. Remove the cookies from the oven and let them cool on the baking sheets for 1 to 2 minutes, then transfer them to wire racks to cool completely. Store the cookies in an airtight container at room temperature for up to 5 days or in the freezer for up to 6 months.

Pictured on p. 154

PUMPKIN OATMEAL RAISIN PECAN COOKIES

My niece loves the flavor of pumpkin and is allergic to cinnamon, so I am always trying to create new pumpkin creations that she might like. When I concocted these, I forgot that she didn't like raisins, but luckily I have a lot of friends who do. The batter is really wet, which creates cake-like cookies. **MAKES 40 TO 42 COOKIES**

1 cup all-purpose flour

1 cup whole wheat flour

1 cup gluten-free rolled oats (not quick cooking)

¾ cup firmly packed dark brown sugar

1 tablespoon baking powder

¼ teaspoon kosher salt

½ teaspoon ground ginger

¾ cup raisins

½ cup unsalted pecans, chopped

¾ cup fresh or canned pumpkin purée

2 tablespoons grapeseed oil

¾ cup fir honey

1½ teaspoons pure vanilla extract

In a large bowl, stir together the all-purpose flour, whole wheat flour, oats, brown sugar, baking powder, salt, ginger, raisins, and pecans. Add the pumpkin purée, grapeseed oil, honey, and vanilla and stir until thoroughly combined. Cover the bowl and refrigerate the batter for at least 1 hour.

Preheat the oven to 350°F. Line two baking sheets with parchment paper.

Place 1 tablespoon of the dough on a prepared baking sheet and flatten it slightly. Repeat this process with the rest of the dough, making sure to space the cookies 2 inches apart.

Transfer the cookies to the oven and bake for 10 minutes, then rotate the baking sheets. Bake for another 10 minutes, or until the cookies are golden on the edges and bottom. Remove the cookies from the oven and let them cool on the baking sheets for 5 minutes, then transfer them to wire racks to cool completely. Store the cookies in an airtight container at room temperature for up to 5 days or in the freezer for up to 6 months.

Pictured on p. 155

LAVENDER DATE BARS

The origins for these bars are found in a Lebanese date cookie recipe I learned at culinary school. They are also an homage to one of my favorite treats: the fig bar. The addition of lavender honey adds a layer of flavor to this rich, buttery cookie bar. 🐝 **MAKES 16 BARS**

FILLING

2½ cups dates, pitted and cut into
  ¼-inch pieces

¼ cup 2% milk

¼ cup unsalted butter

COOKIE DOUGH

3¼ cups all-purpose flour

2 sticks (1 cup) cold unsalted butter,
  cut into ½-inch pieces

¼ cup lavender honey

½ cup 2% milk

To make the filling, combine the dates, milk, and butter in a small saucepan set over medium-low heat, stirring occasionally, for 15 to 20 minutes, or until the dates are softened and start turning into a paste. If the mixture starts to look dry, add more milk and butter, ½ tablespoon of each at a time. Remove the pan from the heat and set it aside to cool.

To make the cookie dough, place the flour, butter, and honey in the bowl of a food processor and pulse until the butter is the size of small peas. With the machine running, add the milk and process until the dough comes together. Turn the dough onto a clean work surface and knead it to make sure it is well blended. Divide the dough into two equal pieces.

Preheat the oven to 350°F. Grease an 8 × 8-inch baking dish with nonstick cooking spray.

Press one half of the dough into the bottom of the baking dish, pressing it out evenly. Add the filling and spread it evenly on top of the dough. Shape the other half of the dough into an 8 × 8-inch square, place it on top of the date mixture, and press firmly.

Transfer the baking dish to the oven and bake for 35 to 40 minutes, or until the cookie is golden brown. Remove the cookie from the oven and let it cool in the dish. Cut it into 16 bars and serve. Store the bars in an airtight container at room temperature for 4 to 5 days.

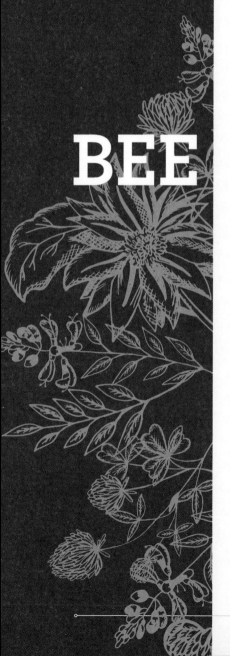

BEE Saucy

CHAPTER 7

Dressings, Marinades, and Sauces

HONEY MUSTARD

This is a basic honey mustard sauce. If you want it a bit spicier, add more mustard. You can use this honey mustard as a dipping sauce for pretzels, as a spread on your favorite sandwich, or as a base for a honey mustard vinaigrette. ❧ **MAKES ¾ CUP**

½ cup wildflower honey
2 tablespoons Dijon mustard

In a small bowl, whisk the honey and mustard together. Transfer the mixture to a small ramekin; cover it and refrigerate until ready to use for up to 2 weeks.

LEMON HONEY VINAIGRETTE

This light vinaigrette works well with mixed greens or on curly kale. ❧ **MAKES 1 ¾ CUPS**

½ cup freshly squeezed lemon juice
½ cup orange blossom honey
½ teaspoon kosher salt
¼ teaspoon freshly ground black pepper
¾ cup olive oil

In a small bowl, whisk together the lemon juice, honey, salt, and pepper. While whisking constantly, slowly stream in the olive oil until it's well emulsified. Store the vinaigrette in an airtight container in the refrigerator for up to 2 weeks.

CRANBERRY ORANGE SAUCE

One of the things I love most about fall is when cranberries become available. Most people think of cranberry sauce as an accompaniment for turkey on Thanksgiving, but I love making a big batch of this sauce to use in dishes throughout the year. Another great thing about cranberries is that you can buy them when they are fresh and freeze them for later. ❧ **MAKES 4 CUPS**

1 navel orange
1 pound fresh or frozen cranberries
1 cup water
½ cup basswood honey

Cut the orange (including the peel) into 8 to 10 pieces. Place the orange pieces in a food processor and pulse until they are finely chopped.

Place the chopped orange, cranberries, and water in a medium saucepan over medium-high heat. Cook, uncovered, for 10 minutes, stirring occasionally, until the cranberries begin to burst. Reduce the heat to low, cover the pan, and cook for another 20 minutes, stirring occasionally. Remove the pan from the heat and stir in the honey. Let the sauce cool. Serve the sauce immediately or store it in an airtight container in the refrigerator for up to 2 weeks or in the freezer for up to 6 months.

NOTE *I like my sauce to be a little tart. I find that if it isn't too sweet, then you can use it in more recipes. If you want it a bit sweeter, add more honey, 1 teaspoon at a time, until it is sweet enough for your taste buds. If you can't find fresh or frozen cranberries, use 8 ounces of dried cranberries instead.*

LEMONGRASS VINAIGRETTE

This vinaigrette can be served with Thai Lemongrass Tofu Salad (page 72), but also try it on your favorite salad or slaw and as an accompaniment to grilled or broiled fish. 🐝
MAKES ABOUT 1 CUP

2 stalks lemongrass, trimmed and minced

2 tablespoons mirin

2 tablespoons sake

2 teaspoons ginger-infused honey

3 tablespoons minced fresh ginger

2 tablespoons tamari

½ cup grapeseed oil

Place the lemongrass, mirin, sake, honey, ginger, and tamari in a blender. Blend on medium speed for 1 minute. With the blender running, slowly add the grapeseed oil until the mixture is well emulsified. Store the vinaigrette in an airtight container in the refrigerator for up to 2 weeks.

MISO VINAIGRETTE

This Asian-inspired vinaigrette is great on mixed greens or drizzled over cooked vegetables. 🐝 **MAKES ABOUT 1½ CUPS**

¼ cup red miso paste

¼ cup rice wine vinegar

¼ cup ginger-infused honey

½ tablespoon tamari

1 tablespoon sesame oil

1 tablespoon freshly squeezed lime juice

¼ cup water

1 clove garlic, sliced

½-inch piece fresh ginger, peeled and sliced

¼ cup grapeseed oil

In a blender, combine the miso paste, vinegar, honey, tamari, sesame oil, lime juice, water, garlic, and ginger. Blend on medium speed for 1 to 2 minutes, or until everything is well incorporated. With the blender running, slowly add the grapeseed oil and blend for 1 minute, or until the mixture is well emulsified. This vinaigrette should be thick. If you want it slightly thinner, add 1 to 2 tablespoons more water. Store the vinaigrette in an airtight container in the refrigerator for up to 2 weeks.

HONEY MUSTARD VINAIGRETTE

If I have any Honey Mustard (page 174) left over, I whisk it into vinaigrette and serve it over mixed greens. It's so simple yet so delicious. 🐝 **MAKES ¾ CUP**

¼ cup wildflower honey

2 tablespoons Dijon mustard

2 tablespoons white wine vinegar

¼ cup grapeseed oil

¼ teaspoon kosher salt

Pinch freshly ground black pepper

In a small bowl, whisk together the honey, mustard, and vinegar. While still whisking, slowly add the grapeseed oil until the mixture is well emulsified. Season with the salt and pepper. Store the vinaigrette in an airtight container in the refrigerator for up to 2 weeks.

FRESH HERB VINAIGRETTE

There is nothing better in the summer than a salad tossed with a vinaigrette packed with fresh herb flavor. The herbs you use are completely up to you—I recommend basil, tarragon, mint, oregano, and/or chives. Serve with your favorite salad or even as an accompaniment to grilled fish. ❧ **MAKES ABOUT 1 CUP**

¼ cup white wine vinegar

1 tablespoon minced shallot

1 clove garlic, minced

1 teaspoon Asheville Bee Charmer's Mint-Infused Honey

1 tablespoon Dijon mustard

½ teaspoon kosher salt

¼ teaspoon freshly ground black pepper

¼ cup roughly chopped fresh flat-leaf parsley leaves

¼ cup olive oil

¼ cup roughly chopped fresh cilantro leaves and stems

¼ cup roughly chopped mixed fresh herb leaves

¼ cup grapeseed oil

1 tablespoon–¼ cup water, if needed

Place the vinegar, shallot, garlic, honey, mustard, salt, pepper, and parsley in a blender. Blend on medium speed for 1 minute. With the blender running, slowly add the olive oil. Add the cilantro and other herbs and blend for 1 minute. With the blender running, slowly add the grapeseed oil until the mixture is well emulsified.

If the vinaigrette seems too thick, add up to ¼ cup of water, 1 tablespoon at a time. Make sure to taste and adjust the seasoning, if needed. Store the vinaigrette in an airtight container in the refrigerator for 3 to 4 days.

BERRY COULIS

Berry coulis can be used on pancakes for breakfast, as an accompaniment for a variety of desserts, or as a topping for your favorite ice cream. ❧ **MAKES ABOUT 1½ CUPS**

12 ounces fresh or frozen blackberries

2 tablespoons blackberry honey

1 tablespoon dry white wine

1 tablespoon freshly squeezed lemon juice

Place all of the ingredients in a blender. Blend on medium speed for 3 to 4 minutes, or until everything is well incorporated. Strain the sauce through a fine-mesh sieve into a bowl or measuring cup. Store the coulis in an airtight container in the refrigerator for up to 7 days or in the freezer for up to 6 months.

NOTE *To make blueberry coulis, use 12 ounces of fresh or frozen blueberries and 2 tablespoons of blueberry honey. To make raspberry coulis, use 12 ounces of fresh or frozen raspberries and 2 tablespoons of raspberry honey. To make strawberry coulis, use 12 ounces of fresh or frozen, hulled strawberries and 2 tablespoons of raspberry honey.*

SESAME SOY HONEY VINAIGRETTE

Drizzle this Asian-inspired vinaigrette on an Asian salad with chicken or fish or over your favorite vegetables. **MAKES ABOUT 1 CUP**

2 tablespoons sesame oil
2 tablespoons ginger-infused honey
¼ cup tamari
¼ cup rice wine vinegar
2 teaspoons roughly chopped fresh ginger
2 teaspoons roughly chopped garlic
¼ cup + 2 tablespoons grapeseed oil

Place the sesame oil, ginger honey, tamari, vinegar, ginger, and garlic in a blender. Blend on medium speed for 1 to 2 minutes, or until smooth. With the blender running, slowly add the grapeseed oil and blend for 1 minute, until the vinaigrette is well emulsified. Store the vinaigrette in an airtight container in the refrigerator for up to 2 weeks.

MISO HONEY GLAZE

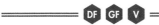

This glaze can be used on chicken, turkey, or fish. **MAKES 1 CUP**

¼ cup sake
¼ cup mirin
¼ cup yellow miso paste
¼ cup acacia honey

In a small bowl, whisk together the sake, mirin, miso, and honey until no lumps remain. Store the glaze in an airtight container in the refrigerator for up to 2 weeks.

HONEY BUTTER

Honey butter is delicious on toast, with biscuits, or on your favorite muffin. I suggest wildflower honey here, but you can use any honey varietal to make the type of honey butter you want. **MAKES ½ CUP**

6 tablespoons unsalted butter, at room temperature
2 tablespoons wildflower honey

In a small bowl, whisk together the butter and honey until well incorporated. Transfer the mixture to a small ramekin, cover it tightly with plastic wrap, and refrigerate until ready to use for up to 7 days.

ASIAN DIPPING SAUCE

This dipping sauce is sweet, spicy, and salty—the perfect complement to your favorite egg roll or spring roll. It is also a great dipping sauce for fish and chicken. **MAKES ABOUT ½ CUP**

¼ cup tamari
1 tablespoon ginger-infused honey
1 tablespoon Asheville Bee Charmer's Ghost Pepper Honey
2 teaspoons minced fresh ginger
½ teaspoon sesame oil
1 green onion, minced

In a small bowl, whisk together all of the ingredients. Store the sauce in an airtight container in the refrigerator for 3 to 4 days.

RHUBARB APPLE SAUCE

This sauce works well with turkey, pork, and potato pancakes. It can also be used as an accompaniment for fruit, ice cream, pound cake, pancakes, and Greek yogurt. ❧ **MAKES ABOUT 2½ CUPS**

½ cup orange blossom honey

¾ cup water

1 tablespoon freshly grated lemon zest

2 large stalks rhubarb, cut into 1-inch pieces (2 cups)

1 large Gala apple, cored, peeled, and cut into 1-inch pieces (1½ cups)

Place the honey, water, lemon zest, rhubarb, and apple in a medium saucepan over medium-high heat and stir well. Bring the mixture to a boil, then reduce the heat to low and simmer, uncovered, for 25 minutes, or until the rhubarb and apple are very soft and mashable.

Blend the sauce in two batches in a blender or use an immersion blender to purée it right in the pan.

Serve the sauce warm, at room temperature, or cold. Store it in an airtight container in the refrigerator for 4 to 5 days or in the freezer for up to 6 months.

BARBEQUE SAUCE

Most barbeque sauce recipes call for it to be cooked over low, slow heat. By using honey rather than sugar, you don't even need to cook this sauce. Make it at least 4 hours and up to 1 day before you plan to use it so that the flavors have a chance to meld together. ❧ **MAKES ABOUT 1¾ CUPS**

1 cup low-sodium organic ketchup

¼ cup buckwheat honey

2 tablespoons Asheville Bee Charmer's Smokin' Hot Honey (chipotle-infused honey)

2 tablespoons apple cider vinegar

1 tablespoon freshly squeezed orange juice

½ tablespoon Worcestershire sauce

2 tablespoons sambal oelek

½ teaspoon ground cumin

½ teaspoon onion powder

½ teaspoon garlic powder

½ teaspoon freshly ground black pepper

Whisk together all the ingredients in a small bowl. Transfer the sauce to an airtight container and store it in the refrigerator for up to 1 month.

SWEET AND SOUR SAUCE

After making your own sweet and sour sauce, you will never buy the bottled variety again. This is a great sauce to use with egg rolls, but you can also use it with pork, chicken, or even meatballs. The trick to making the sauce is to whisk it constantly while it's cooking—otherwise it will get lumpy. ❀ **MAKES ABOUT 1 ¾ CUPS**

1 cup pineapple juice

⅓ cup water

3 tablespoons rice wine vinegar

1 tablespoon tamari

¼ cup basswood honey

¼ cup Asheville Bee Charmer's Firecracker Hot Honey

3 tablespoons cornstarch

Place all the ingredients in a small saucepan and whisk them together until the cornstarch is fully dissolved and blended in. Place the pan over medium-high heat and bring the mixture to a boil, whisking continuously. Once the mixture is boiling, continue stirring the sauce for another 1 to 2 minutes, or until it has thickened.

Remove the pan from the heat and let the sauce cool to room temperature. Transfer the sauce to an airtight container and store it in the refrigerator for up to 1 month.

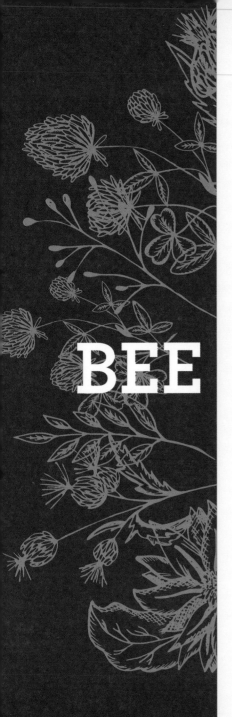

BEE Buzzed

CHAPTER 8

Mocktails and Cocktails

RECIPES BY KIM ALLEN

HONEY SIMPLE SYRUP

Simple syrup is used in many mocktail and cocktail recipes. You can use any type of honey varietal to make your syrup. To prolong its shelf life, add ½ teaspoon of vodka per ounce of simple syrup. 🐝 **MAKES 2 CUPS**

1 cup water

1 cup honey

Heat the water and honey in a small saucepan over medium heat until the honey is completely dissolved. Make sure the mixture does not boil.

Remove the pan from the heat and let the syrup cool to room temperature. Transfer it to an airtight container and store it in the refrigerator for up to 1 month.

INFUSED HONEY SIMPLE SYRUP

There are numerous variations you can make, depending on the honey varietal and fresh herbs you choose. For best results, infuse the syrup for 48 hours. Be adventurous and create your own flavored versions of cocktails! 🐝 **MAKES 2 CUPS**

1 cup water

1 cup honey

¼ cup fresh mint or basil leaves and/or pieces of peeled fresh ginger (you can use any type of herbs or spices that you want to make your own infusions—be creative!)

Heat the water and honey in a small saucepan over medium heat until the honey is completely dissolved. Make sure the mixture does not boil.

Remove the pan from the heat, add the fresh herbs, and let the syrup cool to room temperature. Transfer the syrup to an airtight container and let it sit in the refrigerator for 48 hours.

Strain the herbs from the mixture and return the syrup to the airtight container. Store the syrup in the refrigerator for up to 1 month.

BASIL GIMLET

The gimlet is essentially a gin martini with lime and simple syrup. To really give it a twist, use basil-infused simple syrup. 🐝 **MAKES 1 GIMLET**

¾ ounce freshly squeezed lime juice

¾ ounce clover honey Simple Syrup (page 182)

5 fresh basil leaves, divided

1½ ounces top-shelf gin

Chill a martini glass. Place the lime juice, Simple Syrup, and 4 of the basil leaves in a cocktail shaker. Crush the mixture with a muddler or the back of a spoon to release the basil oils. Add the gin and some ice to the shaker. Cover and shake vigorously for 1 minute.

Strain the mixture into the chilled martini glass. Garnish with the remaining basil leaf and serve.

CHAI SPICED SOUTHERN SWEET TEA

This is a chai twist on an old Southern favorite. ☙ MAKES 1 QUART

4 cups water

3 tablespoons Asheville Bee Charmer's Chai-Infused Honey

3 bags black tea

Bring the water to a boil in a medium saucepan over medium-high heat, then immediately remove the pan from the heat. Add the honey to the boiling water and stir to dissolve. Add the tea bags and let the mixture steep, uncovered, for about 5 minutes.

Remove the tea bags, transfer the tea to an airtight container, and store it in the refrigerator for up to 7 days. Serve the tea hot or chilled over ice.

IRISH COFFEE

Transport yourself to the shores of Ireland on a chilly evening with this simple coffee cocktail. ☙ MAKES 1 SERVING

1 (8-ounce) cup freshly brewed coffee

1 ounce Irish whiskey

2 tablespoons meadowfoam honey

2 tablespoons whipped cream

Pour the coffee into a large mug. Add the whiskey and honey, stirring well until the honey is dissolved. Top with the whipped cream and serve.

SMOKY BLOODY MARY

Sunday mornings and brunch wouldn't be the same without a Bloody Mary. This spicy version will cure whatever ails you! ☙ MAKES 1 BLOODY MARY

2 ounces top-shelf vodka

1 tablespoon Asheville Bee Charmer's Smokin' Hot Honey (chipotle-infused honey)

2 teaspoons Worcestershire sauce

6 ounces tomato vegetable juice

2 teaspoons freshly squeezed lemon juice

Pinch freshly ground black pepper

Celery salt, to taste

2 lemon wedges

1 small skewer with 2 okra pickles and 2 green olives, for garnish

Place the vodka, honey, Worcestershire sauce, tomato vegetable juice, lemon juice, and black pepper in a cocktail shaker. Cover and shake vigorously for 1 to 2 minutes, or until the honey is dissolved. Add ice, cover, and shake until chilled, about 1 minute.

Place the celery salt on a small plate. Rub 1 lemon wedge around the rim of a tall (10- to 12-ounce) glass. Invert the glass onto the celery salt and twist so that the rim is fully covered.

Strain the drink into the glass and add 2 to 3 ice cubes. Garnish with the remaining lemon wedge and the skewer of okra pickles and green olives and serve.

the asheville bee charmer cookbook

LIMONCELLO MARTINI

When you think of classic drinks, a martini always comes to mind. Limoncello adds a touch of sophistication, while the basswood honey adds citrus and light floral overtones to the cocktail. 🐝 **MAKES 1 MARTINI**

2½ ounces top-shelf vodka

1 ounce limoncello liqueur

1 ounce basswood honey Simple Syrup (page 182)

1 twist of lemon peel, for garnish

Chill a martini glass. Combine the vodka, limoncello, and Simple Syrup in a cocktail shaker. Add ice, cover, and shake vigorously for about 1 minute.

Strain the cocktail into the chilled glass. Garnish with the twist of lemon and serve.

ACACIA HONEY-RITA

There is nothing I enjoy more on a hot summer day than a margarita. For a light and delicate twist on an old classic, try this one. 🐝 **MAKES 1 MARGARITA**

1½ ounces top-shelf silver tequila

1 ounce elderflower liqueur

¾ ounce freshly squeezed lime juice

¾ ounce acacia honey Simple Syrup (page 182)

Coarse sea salt, as needed

2 lime wedges

Combine the tequila, elderflower liqueur, lime juice, and Simple Syrup in a cocktail shaker. Add ice, cover, and shake vigorously for 1 minute.

Place the sea salt on a small plate. Rub a lime wedge around the rim of a margarita glass and invert the glass onto the plate of salt. Twist slightly until the edge of the glass is covered with salt.

Strain the margarita into the glass and add 2 to 3 ice cubes. Garnish with the remaining lime wedge and serve.

SWEET BEE BOURBON COCKTAIL

Bourbon cocktails are a staple in the South. To make this even more interesting, infuse the wildflower simple syrup with ginger or thyme. 🐝 **MAKES 1 COCKTAIL**

1½ ounces top-shelf bourbon

½ teaspoon wildflower honey Simple Syrup (page 182)

6 ounces ginger beer or ginger ale

Mix the bourbon and Simple Syrup in a cocktail shaker. Add ice, cover, and shake vigorously for 1 minute.

Strain the mixture into a short 10- to 12-ounce cocktail glass filled with ice. Top with the ginger beer or ginger ale and serve.

MOJITO

DF **GF** **V**

A mojito is incredibly refreshing in the summer, but it can transport you to the island getaway in your mind any time of the year. ❦ **MAKES 1 MOJITO**

1½ ounces mint-acacia honey Infused Simple Syrup (page 182)

¾ ounce freshly squeezed lime juice

7 fresh mint leaves, divided

2 ounces top-shelf white rum

6–8 ounces club soda

1 lime wedge, for garnish

Combine the Simple Syrup, lime juice, and 5 mint leaves in a cocktail shaker. Crush the mixture with a muddler or the back of a spoon to release the mint oils. Add the rum and some ice. Cover and shake vigorously for 1 minute.

Strain the mixture into a tall (12- to 14-ounce) glass. Top with the club soda. Garnish with the 2 remaining mint leaves and the lime wedge and serve.

Acknowledgements

Thanks to Jillian Kelly and Kim Allen for allowing me to become the Asheville Bee Charmer's "Waggle Dancer." To Chefs Michel Coatrieux, Pierre Pollin, and Peggy Ryan for inspiring me as a chef, informing my technique, teaching me the importance of cooking from the heart, and encouraging my creativity in the kitchen. To Elena Marre and Anastasia Laborde for sharing their knowledge about healthy vegetarian cooking. To Chef Tom Leavitt for sharing his culinary knowledge and technique. Thanks to Angela Garbot for her photography skills and creativity. Thanks to Jill Houk for sharing her culinary knowledge and technique as well as her food styling expertise. And, finally, many thanks to all my family and friends for willingly eating and giving me feedback on the recipes.

APPENDIX A

Recipes by Honey Varietal

VARIETAL	RECIPE	PAGE
ACACIA HONEY	Acacia Honey-rita	184
	Apricot Glazed Chicken Kebabs	107
	Caponata	132
	Chocolate Pistachio Baklava	160
	Honey Mustard Glazed Halibut	92
	Lemon Ricotta Blueberry Pancakes	36
	Miso Honey Glaze	177
	Miso Honey Glazed Salmon	94
	Mojito	185
	Tropical Oat, Nut, and Chocolate Bars	54
BASSWOOD HONEY	Brie, Cranberry, and Almond Phyllo Cups	44
	Cranberry Orange Sauce	174
	Curried Chicken Salad	66
	ELT	89
	Grilled Cheese with Cranberry and Ghost Pepper	96
	Limoncello Martini	184
	Roasted Pork Tenderloin with Apricot Chutney	113
	Sweet and Sour Sauce	179
	Thai Lemongrass Tofu Salad	72
	Turkey, Cranberry, and Honey Herb Cream Cheese Sandwich	102
BLACKBERRY HONEY	Berry Chia Seed Pudding	162
	Berry Coulis	176
	Blackberry Mead Poached Pears with Honey Ricotta	163
	French Toast with Berry Coulis	32

the asheville bee charmer cookbook

Recipes by Dietary Restriction

RECIPE	PAGE	DAIRY FREE	GLUTEN FREE	VEGETARIAN
Acacia Honey-rita	184	●	●	●
Amaranth, Nut, and Seed Bars	34		●	●
Apple and Sage Buckwheat	141	●	●	●
Apple Cinnamon Walnut Cake with Chai Honey Glaze	168			●
Apple Lavender Muffins	31			●
Apple Parsnip Soup	70	●	●	●
Apricot Glazed Chicken Kebabs	107	●	●	
Asian Dipping Sauce	177	●	●	●
Asian Duck Cigars	62			
Asian Edamame Burgers	123	●	●	●
Asian Turkey Lettuce Cups	114	●	●	
Barbeque Chicken	111	●	●	
Barbeque Sauce	178	●	●	●
Basil Gimlet	182	●		●
Bee Pollen Nut Brittle	47		●	●
Berry Chia Seed Pudding	162	●	●	●
Berry Coulis	176	●	●	●
Black Bean Brownies	159	●		●
Blackberry Mead Poached Pears with Honey Ricotta	163		●	●
Bolivian Baked Buckwheat	127		●	●
Braised Garbanzos and Chicken Sausage	90	●	●	
Breakfast Bread Pudding	39			
Brie, Cranberry, and Almond Phyllo Cups	44			●

RECIPE	PAGE	DAIRY FREE	GLUTEN FREE	VEGETARIAN
Cabbage, Gorgonzola, and Candied Walnut Empanadas	58			●
Candied Orange Olive Oil Almond Cake	165	●	●	●
Candied Walnuts	55	●	●	●
Caponata	132	●	●	●
Carrot Freekeh	133	●		●
Carrot Orange Sunflower Date Muffins	33	●		●
Chai Pumpkin Pie	164		●	●
Chai Spiced Southern Sweet Tea	183	●	●	●
Chipotle Honey Marinated Skirt Steak	99	●	●	
Chocolate Avocado Mousse	150	●	●	●
Chocolate Hazelnut Pinwheels	157			●
Chocolate Honey Almond No-Bake Granola Bars	49		●	●
Chocolate Pistachio Baklava	160			●
Citrus Spinach Salad	79	●	●	●
Corn Chowder	83		●	●
Cranberry Orange Sauce	174	●	●	●
Curried Chicken Salad	66	●	●	
Curried Squash Soup with Spiced Pumpkin Seeds	78	●	●	●
Duck à l'Orange	119	●	●	
Eggplant Parmesan Stacks	131		●	●
ELT	89	●		●
Everyday Granola	28	●	●	●
French Toast with Berry Coulis	32			●
Fresh Herb Vinaigrette	176	●	●	●
Ginger Lime Shrimp	118	●	●	
Ginger Orange Mashed Sweet Potatoes	140		●	●
Grilled Cheese with Cranberry and Ghost Pepper	96			●
Grilled Indian Fruit Salad with Spiced Yogurt	151		●	●
Healthy Garbage Salad	71	●	●	●
Hearty Greens Slaw	85	●	●	●

the asheville bee charmer cookbook

RECIPE	PAGE	DAIRY FREE	GLUTEN FREE	VEGETARIAN
Miso Honey Glaze	177	●	●	●
Miso Honey Glazed Salmon	94	●	●	
Miso Vinaigrette	175	●	●	●
Mojito	185	●	●	●
Moroccan Carrot Soup	82		●	●
Moroccan Chicken	112	●	●	
Moroccan Couscous	137			●
Peanut Butter Chocolate Chip Cookies	169			●
Piñaprese	80			●
Pork Adobo	110	●	●	
Pulled Pork	106	●	●	
Pumpkin Leek Soup	76	●	●	●
Pumpkin Oatmeal Raisin Pecan Cookies	170	●		●
Ragin' Asian Ribs	91	●	●	
Rhubarb Apple Sauce	178	●	●	●
Roasted Beets with Honey Chive Goat Cheese	84		●	●
Roasted Honey Glazed Chicken	109	●	●	
Roasted Pear, Blue Cheese, and Walnut Phyllo Bites	48			●
Roasted Pineapple Chai Sorbet	161	●	●	●
Roasted Pork Tenderloin with Apricot Chutney	113	●	●	
Roasted Spaghetti Squash with Herbs	134		●	●
Roasted Squash, Quinoa, Cranberry, and Pecan Salad	69	●	●	●
Roasted Turkey Breast with Rhubarb Apple Glaze	122	●	●	
Rosemary Polenta Cake	148		●	●
Sesame Beef and Asparagus Salad	74	●		
Sesame Crusted Tuna	101	●	●	
Sesame Soy Honey Vinaigrette	177	●	●	●
Shiitake and Cabbage Egg Rolls	57	●		●
Smoky Bloody Mary	183	●		●

INDEX

ABOUT THE AUTHOR

Carrie Schloss earned a degree in finance from Miami University and an MBA in finance and international business from the University of Chicago. After a successful career in international investments, she shifted gears to pursue a lifelong dream of working in the culinary industry. She graduated from the culinary school at Kendall College and currently works as a personal chef and culinary consultant specializing in creating recipes for those with specific dietary needs. She has developed recipes for *Let's Dish*, a cooking show on the Live Well television network, and for the past six years, she has taught cooking classes for kids and adults at The Kids' Table, Now We're Cooking, and nonprofit organizations such as Common Threads, Purple Asparagus, and Chicago Lights Urban Farm Cooking. She has known Queen Bee Kim for over 30 years and Queen Bee Jillian for over 20 years. *The Asheville Bee Charmer Cookbook* is her first cookbook. She lives in Wilmette, Illinois.

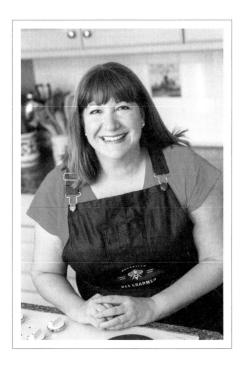